DOUGLAS WAGEMANN II

Enlighten Me

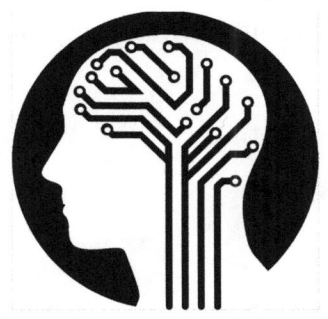

First published by Virtues of Mental Health 2019

Copyright © 2019 by Douglas Wagemann II

All rights reserved. No part of this publication may be reproduced, stored or transmitted in any form or by any means, electronic, mechanical, photocopying, recording, scanning, or otherwise without written permission from the publisher. It is illegal to copy this book, post it to a website, or distribute it by any other means without permission.

Douglas Wagemann II asserts the moral right to be identified as the author of this work.

The information in this book is for educational purposes only and does not replace the need for assessment and treatment performed by a licensed trained professional in mental health. Education in this book is geared towards informing the public and is in no way personalized treatment. If you are thinking or intending on hurting yourself or hurting other people, ALWAYS call 911 or go to your nearest emergency department for immediate help.

First edition

ISBN: 978-1-7341628-0-6

This book was professionally typeset on Reedsy.
Find out more at reedsy.com

To Shawna,

Your life was full of beauty and turmoil, love and heinousness, yet we experienced this reality together. Always know that we were trying our best with what we knew, what we thought was best, and with what resources we had. I hope to help others who experience the same realities we did. This work is dedicated to you, my sister.

Shawna Lynn Wagemann Jensen

1975-2018

Contents

Preface	ii
INTRODUCTION: WHY DID I PICK UP THIS BOOK?	1
THE DIAGNOSIS	7
MOOD DISORDERS	17
PSYCHOSIS DISORDERS	36
PERSONALITY DISORDERS	52
EATING DISORDERS	72
PTSD AND OTHER MENTAL DISORDERS	80
THE MEDICATIONS	89
THE PSYCHOTHERAPIES	150
SUBSTANCE USE AND ADDICTION	187
SUBSTANCE USE AND ADDICTION TREATMENT	219
UNIQUE POPULATIONS AND CONSIDERATIONS	237
A TRAUMA MANIFESTO	256
CONCLUSION	271
RESOURCES	274
REFERENCES	277
About the Author	287

Preface

MENTAL HEALTH PROFESSIONAL TYPES

Medical Doctor: Medical doctors are probably the most recognized of healthcare professionals. Medical Doctors (MD or DO) go to medical school after their bachelor's degree for 4 years after which they do a residency in their specialty, which can range from 2-6 years. In mental health, you will see psychiatrists, family medicine doctors, and pediatric medicine doctors who diagnose and prescribe mental illnesses. *Other terms: Primary Care Provider (PCP), physician, Generalist, Doctor of Osteopathy (DO)*

Psychiatrist: a psychiatrist is a medical doctor who has gone through medical school like any other medical doctor. They then go into a psychiatry residency that specializes their training in psychiatry. They diagnose mental illnesses, prescribe psychiatric medications, and some provide psychotherapy and electroconvulsive therapy (ECT). *PsychIAtrist tends to be mixed up with psychOLOgist. See next for psychologist. Other terms: "shrink"*

Nurse Practitioner: a nurse practitioner is an advanced practice nurse, meaning they have at least a master's degree, a nursing license, and a specialized certification in being a nurse practitioner. Nurse practitioners can diagnose, prescribe, and order tests like a medical doctor. Psychiatric mental health nurse practitioners (PMHNP) specialize in psychiatry and diagnose mental illnesses, prescribe psychiatric medications, and some provide psychotherapy. Family nurse practitioners will also treat uncomplicated mental illnesses. *Other terms: APRN, NP*

Physician Assistant: a physician assistant (PA) is a provider who specializes in diagnosing, prescribing, and ordering treatments. Their training is along the "medical model," meaning it most fits into the medical school curriculum. Physician assistants tend to be seen in primary care or in highly specialized fields, such as orthopedic surgery, dermatology, etc. There are few who specialize in psychiatry, but they do exist out there and are fully qualified to diagnose and prescribe medications. Their degree requirements are also a masters level degree. *Other terms: PA, physician extender*

Clinical Psychologist: a clinical psychologist is a doctorate educated professional who is highly specialized in psychotherapy, mental illness diagnosis, and specialized testing for brain disorders. There are two degree types you will see, the *PhD* and the *PsyD*. Both are fully qualified and provide excellent psychotherapy and diagnostics. The difference is the focus, where the PhD tends to be more research focused, and the PsyD tends to be more clinical focused. They are licensed. *Other terms: therapist, "shrink,", psychotherapist, neuropsychologist*

Marriage and Family Therapist: **Marriage and family therapists (MFT)** specialize in therapy that generally is focused on family and relationship dynamics. The degree requirement is a masters degree and required internship hours to get licensure. While specializing in relationship dynamics, you will see MFTs do individual therapy and group therapy. *Other terms: therapist, psychotherapist*

Licensed Professional Clinical Counselor: a licensed professional clinical counselor (LPCC) specializes in psychotherapy and is geared more to the individual, although they are trained in group therapies as well. LPCC's complete internship hours to receive licensure. LPCCs are well rounded educated in many therapy types and are very commonly seen in all states with the exception of California, where you will see more MFTs. *Other terms:*

therapist, LPC

Social Worker: a social worker is a person of many hats. Social workers training is geared towards resources and support. Many times you see social workers in the government, working for child protective services, or working in hospitals to help obtain resources for patients. Social workers are approved to provide psychotherapy, and some do solely specialize in psychotherapy. Like MFTs and LPCCs, social workers have a masters degree and are required to do internship hours in order to be licensed. *Other terms: LCSW, therapist, associate clinical social worker (ASW)*

Certified Alcohol Drug Counselor: typically seen in rehabs, certified alcohol drug counselors have a certificate that specializes in addiction counseling. Skills include crisis management, skill, and coping development, and understanding of the different types of substances abused. Some have "lived experience," meaning that they have a substance abuse history and are in recovery. There are many names for the certificate and is largely depends on the state certifying body for the naming of these professionals. *Other terms: drug/alcohol counselor, counselor, certified addiction specialist, addiction counselor*

1

INTRODUCTION: WHY DID I PICK UP THIS BOOK?

"The thing that keeps someone living is a sense of future."
-**Stephen Fry**

Who will find this book useful?

Mental illness – it's a word that, for some with it, is as comfortable and ingrained as breathing. These people tend to live in a world where their mental illness or that of their loved one is an everyday occurrence and reality. For others, and I might dare say most, the word mental illness brings on discomfort and distress that can be similar to topics like death or violence. It is the unfamiliar, the alien, the "person who was okay and now is different." For those who recently got a new mental illness diagnosis or if you have a loved one who is recently diagnosed, the event can be devastating. The five years, ten years, and maybe 50-years plan may seem destroyed, and uncertainty hits like a brick wall. Suddenly, the questions begin to flood the brain, "what is going on?", "is my loved one ever going to be 'normal'?", "Is this going to be forever?", "what changes are going to happen because of this?", and a whole lot of other related thoughts. These questions are, of course, normal and expected. It is no more different than when someone gets diagnosed with any other chronic disease. Yet, mental illness has a component to it that is not like other medical diagnoses. One that is shriveled with stigma, misunderstanding, fear, and coupled with a system that is considered to be one of the most broken systems in the entire U.S. healthcare system.

This book is for people who have been recently diagnosed with a mental illness and for those whose loved one has recently been diagnosed with a mental illness. This book can also be for seasoned people with mental illness who want to gain some more understanding of their illness, along with treatment options. Clinicians and professionals in the field of mental health may also find this book useful to add depth to their knowledge base. In my years as a psychiatric nurse and nurse practitioner, I have counseled thousands of families who can be, at times, more distressed than their actual family members with mental illness. To receive the news of a mental illness diagnosis has a big impact, but to try and figure out the mental health system is nothing short of frustrating, disheartening, and the number one reason for the hopelessness and helplessness that so many experience. These factors all lead up to what the mental health community sees and experiences with their families. And we are not done yet. This all can be very overwhelming, but then add on when a person with mental illness doesn't want to engage with treatment, and maybe there are substances involved that complicate the whole picture of treatment and engagement with the mental health system. The lack of insight that can be seen in some mental illnesses will be discussed later in this book, but for those who are facing it; this can be one of the most despairing of all feelings. What do you do if you provide all the treatment and help a person could ever ask for, only for them to turn it down, state they are not ill, and maybe even become agitated and break a relationship with you? Unfortunately, this is all too common and experienced by the person with mental illness, the family, and mental health staff.

INTRODUCTION: WHY DID I PICK UP THIS BOOK?

The goal of this book is to help provide some clarity with different mental illnesses, addictions, and their treatments. This book is not designed to fix the mental health system or to diagnose yourself or a loved one. My hope is that this book will be an aid and educational resource into the different types of mental illnesses, their treatments, and the mental health system. Clarity and learning can be an empowering and effective means of decision making for you and your loved one. Having a good grasp of the understanding of any mental illness and ways to navigate the mental health system will always be more advantageous than walking in the dark. It is my goal that you will gain insight, clarity, and vigor to be able to advocate and gain a new depth of mental health understanding and options pertaining to treatment.

Cheers to that.

Stigma

Mental illness is incredibly isolating. Anyone who has experienced mental illness knows exactly what I am talking about. You feel like an alien in a world where everyone "seems normal" and where "they don't seem to get you." This leads people who are suffering to hide in the dark, to pretend, and live in a world where their suffering is not being understood or acknowledged. It's no wonder they can further decompensate and go into a spiral leading to potential inpatient hospitalization. We all have our breaking point. Even more unfortunate is the immense and insidious stigma around mental illness. Stigma in mental illness can be experienced from strangers, family and friends, healthcare professionals, and with actual sufferers of mental illness. At times, people with mental illness may have the biggest stigma towards mental illness as they fight with both shame and a longing to try and belong with "normal" society by either denying or ridiculing others for the very thing that they are suffering from.

Why stigma? Why are so many people adverse to those with mental illness? You could spend a whole Ph.D. education on just stigma as it is incredibly complicated and multifaceted. Breaking it down, we see that our human nature and instincts can play a role in the formation of separating from others and further stigmatizing them. Humans tend to distance themselves from all things that are "unknown" or "unpredictable". "This can be dangerous" is what our instincts naturally tell us. "Thus, I shouldn't associate with it or be near it" is the general result of those initial feelings. The act of stigmatizing is a way to separate oneself from whoever they are stigmatizing. It creates an "us vs. them" mentality that gives the person comfort, and self-esteem boosts that are very reinforcing to perform again. We are avoidant of suffering, and we live in a world where we want to "see no evil, hear no evil, and do no evil," which sadly makes humans tend to turn away from human suffering, especially when it is complex, misunderstood, and foreign.

The complexity and subjective expression of mental illness also complicate matters for the general public. Remember, humans love and cherish predictability. One goes to shop and has a general expectation not to be yelled at, or maybe feel uncomfortable due to behaviors they are not used to. Mental Illness is that general shift from what the general public "expects and wants" for their normal well-being. Unfortunately, instead of embracing those who are suffering, they will tend to avoid and instill the harsh separating words of "crazy" or "insane," which will further alienate the individual with mental illness. The brain, in itself, is the most complicated organ in the human body. No person is alike in genetic makeup, personality, and behaviors. Each of us expresses ourselves in our own individualities in part from the complexity of our brain's ability to be so adaptable, so expressive, and so complex. Because of this, afflictions with mental illness will lead to an array of signs and symptoms that *may* resemble a mental illness diagnosis, but it will be almost present within the individuality of that person who has the mental illness.

What does this do? It makes categorizing, objective measures, recognition, and embracement very challenging and, once again, vague. People don't like this, so they tend to live in a world of misunderstanding and have great difficulty separating the "illness" from the "person". The easiest thing for the brain to do is to simply say "it's the person, they are crazy" as a whole. They then tend to throw people with mental illness into a "bucket" of "what people with mental illness are," which of course has the person who is suffering social phobia to the person with severe mental illness who is chronically homeless and even a murderer who was high on drugs and acting oddly, or the "crazy" case of Jeffrey Dahmer who had schizotypal and borderline personality features. A person who is suffering from mental illness, whether minimal symptoms to full severe mental illness, has to contend with this in public. The pressure to not fall in that bucket is incredible as we generally want to belong and be connected with humanity. Families face the same struggle as they tend to not tell others about a loved one who is suffering from mental illness. This is both to not risk stigma for their loved one but also for themselves. It tends to be far easier for those with mental illness to try and hide their suffering to appease the public and be rewarded with a feeling of belonging.

We have a long way to go with raising awareness and activating stigma reducing programs. 1 in 5 persons have a diagnosable mental illness, and it will not simply go away by "wishing" or "ignoring" it away. Stigma Reduction programs have been instigated in the United States and generally have been an abysmal failure. At best, there was a moderate reduction in believing that mental illness has a biological component like any other medical condition, but there is no reduction in beliefs that people with mental illness are "dangerous" or "crazy". Interestingly enough, research shows that the best stigma buster is simply a personal meeting and learning of a person's mental illness. We see this so much in history. So many societal fears in history were mostly from a lack of exposure. Once perceived opponents got to know each other, the separating walls dropped, and humanity was seen in both. This makes sense once again with our biology from above. Yet, we have the tendency to do the exact opposite which provides a barrier to stigma reduction. We in the mental health community have an uphill battle with the general public, sadly. To gain understanding and acceptance of mental illness is challenging and unfortunately tends to lead to worse suffering from feelings of "not being strong enough" or "being defective". It contributes to our broken mental health system and the challenges of being taken seriously. It wasn't until the Affordable Care Act that mental health services were given mandatory coverage like any other ailment. This spells out to people that mental illness is not the same as physical illnesses and is actually deserving of fewer treatment options. We know that quality of mind, happiness, and sanity are incredibly important for our quality of life, maybe even more so than many other physical illnesses.

This book will hopefully not only provide you or your loved one with information on mental illness but also serve as an eye-opener to the status quo of the mental health community. To those in the mental health community, this all makes tremendous sense. It is always important to remember that humans tend to think simple answers to complex experiences, and if their answers are not satisfied, they will avoid or reject the complexity with even more simplicity, or by distancing from the unknown.

2

THE DIAGNOSIS

"Diagnosis is not the end, but the beginning of practice"
- Martin H. Fischer MD

Mental illness diagnosis — a complex and complicated (are we picking up a theme here?) term that can mean so many different things. For the newly diagnosed, this is truly frightening, but it can also be very liberating, "Finally, there is a name and understanding to these strong emotions or thoughts I've been having!". For many loved ones, it can spell a recipe for a feeling of being lost at sea, shock, lost, and confusion. This chapter is for the education and recognition of different mental illnesses. Included are the diagnostic criteria along with general patterns and recognition tips for the person or loved one suffering from mental illness. Understanding the illness can give profound empowerment and help prevent furthering and worsening episodes. Furthermore, it should be noted that the diagnosis of mental illness gives us guidance. Learning the individual and how they present the signs and symptoms is the first step to providing care and advocating for proper treatment.

Basics of Diagnosing

The diagnostics and naming of mental illnesses have changed dramatically from its origins in the 19th century. Schizophrenia used to be seen as *Dementia Proxemia* and had broad symptoms, which are now more narrowed and categorized as subtypes. In the United States, diagnostics of mental illnesses utilize the famous (or infamous) *Diagnostics and Statistical Manual of Mental Disorders (DSM)*. Its first edition was created in 1952 to provide a categorized and standardized method of diagnosing mental illnesses in the United States. The DSM is now in its 5th edition and has changed dramatically from the 1st edition. Its drastic changes across editions, unfortunately, can fuel the confusion by the public about what mental illness is and what it isn't. The DSM is the standard in psychiatry and is generally seen to be an authority in mental illness diagnostics. It is ridiculed with controversy by many people in the general public and professionally, and probably with some deserving. Homosexuality was seen as a "sociopathic" personality disturbance and remained a "disorder" until 1973. You can also imagine the detrimental and failed therapies given to many homosexual people and the torture of going through such therapies.

Nonetheless, the team of specialists in psychiatry who panel and go through revising the DSM in each edition are not evil or ill-intended. Culture and "norms" play into every human, and with that will come misconceptions and errors in any formation of diagnostics. The panels are in all senses, doing the best they can with the resources and research available to them. They have every intention to get this right and to make it clearer and clearer, if not more so than others in the mental health community. It is referred colloquially as the *Bible of Psychiatry*, which is not what it is by any means. One of the criticisms of the DSM is that it makes the clinician try to fit the patient into the diagnosis. This is a bad practice by clinicians due to the reality of our complexities and in more regard, isn't fair to the patient. The DSM should always be referred to as a guide to diagnostics. But remember, humans like certainty, so many clinicians will try to fit the picture exactly. Regardless of our thoughts of the DSM, we are stuck with it in the mental health system, so it is a manual we need to learn and be content with.

Internationally, the *International Classification of Diseases (ICD)* is mostly utilized as the mental illness diagnostic manual. In its 10th edition, the ICD-10, as it's called now, is interestingly created in the United States and is copyrighted by the World Health Organization (WHO). The ICD-10 includes both mental illnesses and all other medical illnesses, unlike the DSM, which is solely mental illnesses. The ICD-10 original intent is to provide an international coding for diagnoses for billing and research purposes. They have criteria for diagnoses but not to the level of the DSM-5. There is work to correlate DSM-5 diagnostics to ICD-10 coding to make it more uniform, but this has been long discussed with minimal progression as of 2019.

Diagnosing in mental health remains mostly subjective — meaning that a diagnosis is based on what the diagnoser sees and receives from the person. This can be challenging to make consistent across the throngs of providers who diagnose. This is a difference in mental health compared to most medical conditions, which will have components of subjective data but also objective data such as labs or imaging. As a provider, I can hear the symptoms of upper right area pain, worsening after eating, increased gas production, burning, and sharp. Now I may be thinking peptic ulcer, but another clinician may be thinking cholecystitis (inflamed gallbladder). In most regards, we are both hitting the spot when looking at subjective data. Is one of us worse than the other? Who is wrong at this point? We are both doing the best with subjective data and the given criteria of medical diagnoses with the given symptoms. Now, we decide to order an ultrasound and some basic labs. Our results show increased C-reactive protein (signs of inflammation) and an increase in white blood cells (response to inflammation). The ultrasound shows us some nice thickening of the gallbladder wall. Now, we both agree that this is cholecystitis and cholecystectomy is needed right away. In mental health, we would still be at the subjective data stage and basically stuck there.

This is a judgment call as it is related to perspective. What is it that I'm seeing and being told and what is the diagnosis that has the highest probability of being correct? Science and research have not gotten to the point of another diagnosis of medical illnesses in mental illness. There are no imaging or labs that tell me that someone has bipolar disorder or schizophrenia. In time, we all hope that science will further give clinicians the tools to gain objective data to support and narrow our mental illness diagnosis. Until then, we are stuck with the current methods that can create more confusion and less "buy-in" by people with mental illnesses who already may feel that they don't have a mental illness.

It isn't uncommon for a person with mental illness who has been in the system for years to have had many diagnoses over the years. They may have started with major depressive disorder in 1982, then later had a manic episode in 1989, so now a bipolar disorder. Then in 1995, when having another episode of mania, the person had hallucinations. Well, now the person is diagnosed with bipolar disorder with psychotic features. But wait, did he just tell me that he had had these voices his whole life, even when he was in a stable mood, but didn't tell anyone until me? Well, now he has schizoaffective disorder, bipolar type. You can see the mess of how the diagnoses have changed over time based on the subjective data given to the clinicians. Were they wrong at the point they diagnosed? Not particularly, they gave a diagnosis that was meeting the criteria of the subjective data. The treatments they then provided most likely helped the person. But you can see how this person, when asked what they have as a mental illness diagnosis, may say, "I have a depressive disorder, I'm bipolar, I'm schizophrenic and psychotic," and you can see why he would name all those. This is one of the challenges with diagnosing. The brain is not categorized into criteria. There is much overlap with the different disorders that need to be taken into account. Unfortunately, for the general public, this massive confusing and misunderstanding makes them believe that mental health treatment is a scam and that those with mental illness don't really have a mental illness because "it's subjective." Diagnosing in mental health is a work in progress and a rather prolonged event, it takes time and continuous interviewing and contact with clinicians to provide enough history and information to rule out certain disorders, which do have overlap. This is why I tend to tell families to try and not ruminate on the "mental illness diagnosis." It does provide some clarity and a name to what's going, but it may not be the say all. We will discuss more about treatments and how many treatments can line up with diagnoses based on signs and symptoms presented.

Where did this mental illness come from?

This is a question often faced when one hears about a newly diagnosed mental illness. "Does it run in the family?" "Is it because of drugs?" or "I am so baffled on how this just showed up." The onset of mental illness can be a slow progression or can be very abrupt. Mental illnesses have had a tremendous amount of research involved in their origins and onsets. In general, there is a consistent consensus that mental illnesses have a genetic basis whereby it runs in families. "But there is no mental illness in my family?". This may be true, but at times when families look back in their generation line, they can find a father, a grandparent, biological uncle who had what was maybe an undiagnosed mental illness. "Dad was a big gambler and had alcoholism," well maybe it was undiagnosed bipolar disorder. Does this mean that if my mother has a major depression disorder that I will be getting it? Not necessarily. Genetics are a funny thing. Genes are inherited from your biological parents. When you get your genes, they give a code to start building structures, almost like a blueprint. They are built based upon the blueprints of the inherited parent. When building structures, the affected genes can build structures (in the brain) that have structural and regulation vulnerabilities. This increases the risk but is not direct absolute causation to mental illness. Because we are all individualistically unique, people are born with these combinations of brain structures that have a unique combination of abilities to make and regulate the brain chemicals that are important for our wellbeing. So, people that have mental illness have bad brains?

Inherently not at all! I live in California. We are the land of shake and bake, and we get high heat and earthquakes. Earthquakes can be devastating and challenging. Minnesota doesn't get earthquakes and, if so, incredibly rare and minimal. Does this mean that California is "disordered" or "bad" because of its propensity to get earthquakes? Not at all. It's simply how California's geography sets the conditions and vulnerabilities that lead to increases in earthquakes. And by the way, Minnesota has its own challenges. Their winters are tough and challenging. Once again, it is the conditions of that area of Minnesota that give it more propensity to have terrible winters. We are like California and Minnesota (or anywhere else). We have our unique strengths and unique vulnerabilities because of factors we cannot control. Are these areas inherently bad or wrong? Not even. The things we can control is how we behave to help lessen the intensity of these vulnerabilities, such as building codes, emergency supplies, warning systems, etc. This doesn't take the vulnerability away completely but mitigates the severity and gives us better chances of maintaining well-being. Genetics is only one piece of the pie though, and there are other factors involved that can contribute to the onset of mental illness.

The environment plays a significant role in the formation of mental illnesses. Life for any human is stressful; for some, it is more than others. Our bodies endure stresses on a daily basis, and for the most part, our body is pretty good at resiliency and being able to take on stressors. There are times in life when maybe a stressor completely overwhelms the regulation of the brain. This could be anything from your first break up, a grandparent dying, or maybe mom and dad are getting divorced. These can be critical times for the brain, and the brain needs to be functioning at optimum condition for the person to get through this. Trauma, either physical, emotional, sexual or neglect, wreaks havoc on the brain. Whether one event, such as sexual assault, or many "micro" traumas, such as repeated "whoopings" or being told you are not good enough, the brain changes in response to these massive stressors on the brain. The "fear" response part of the brain starts to dominate the other brain structures that deal with decision making, impulse control, and the ability to relate to others. You put these types of stressors into a brain that is genetically vulnerable, and you may have created the perfect recipe for the onset for mental illness.

Understanding the genetic and environment roles in increasing the risk of mental illness is the first step to understanding why and how a mental illness come about. The *Diathesis Stress Model* is the general consensus in the mental health community for giving some clarity for the onset of mental illnesses. In its simple form, the *Diathesis Stress Model* states that the brain is created by inherited genes that have vulnerabilities in its structure and function. When environmental stressors occur, the environment "unlocks" the dysregulation from the structural vulnerabilities in the brain which leads to the expression of the mental illness. Does this mean that a person can have genetically built structural parts in the brain but not a mental illness? Yes, this is possible and does occur. The example I do give to my students and families is as follows: a car factory (genes) has the blueprints to start building a car (brain). The car is built and functions pretty well, but unbeknownst to the blueprints and builders, there is a hose that isn't secured tightly enough. The car (brain) drives and handles well for the first 3-4 years without any issues. The owner is not aware of the hose that isn't secured enough, but it is tight enough not to cause any issues. Then, one day, the car is pushed harder than it ever has been. The owner is late to work and is flooring the accelerator and pushing the engine ever so hard to get to work fast. This pushing of the engine by the accelerator (stressor) finally provides enough pressure to pop that hose right off, and now the car is not functioning properly and is now noticeable. This is why mental illnesses tend to have onsets later in life than right away after a person is born. You can see how a person can experience the same stressor as another person, but maybe that person doesn't have the genetically built vulnerable structures like the other has, which is why one person will develop the mental illness, but the other person will not. One of the biggest frustrations is when a stranger states, "Well, I've been through much worse, and I'm okay." This is a failure to understand how the body works. We all do not have the same structures that operate at the same levels at the same time. The brain has vulnerabilities through genetics just like a person may have vulnerabilities to diabetes due to their mother having diabetes. There are times when the person who has a sudden onset of mental illness doesn't have any "perceivable" stressors going on, which shows that the brain is even more vulnerable and sensitive to the environment. Once there is some understanding of the genetics and environmental factors involved in mental illness, many find a pattern or begin to understand why person A got this, and person B did not.

General Onset

The *Diathesis Stress Model* gives some understanding and clarity to the onset of mental illness, but when does the average person start to show mental illness symptoms? The truth is at any age, but we do have data that shows that most mood disorders (depression, bipolar) and thought disorders (schizophrenia, other psychotic disorders) tend to onset between the ages of 18-26. There are multitudes of ideas and reasons for this age group to have a high prevalence of mental illness onset. For starters, the brain of a child and early adolescents is incredibly fluid and resilient. This is due to it needing to develop quickly and efficiently to the different growing stages. Once a person hits the 18-21 range, the brain becomes less fluid and more solid in its structures. The more solidified and rigid the brain is, the harder a stressor hits it simply because it is not as resilient or reactive to the stressor as it was during child development. Second, for anyone in their adulthood, how were your years between 18 and 26? If you say it was the easiest years of your life, consider yourself lucky. This is a time for the young adult to move away from the nest, to take on the responsibilities of an adult (education, marriage, children, debt, etc.), and to start making big decisions in life. This is generally a very hard transition in life and, some would argue, the most challenging of life transitions. Put these new and difficult stressors on a brain that is now less resilient and vulnerable to mental illness, and you know you have a perfect storm recipe. As stated above, the onset can occur at any age, but the tendency is most rampant in this age range.

Sadly, I cannot tell you how many high school seniors who are in their last quarter of high school come to me with first-episode psychosis, or panic disorder, or suicide attempts. Big things are happening for these people, graduating and stress with school, where do I go next? College? Job? Will I ever see my friends again as they are leaving for different schools? The comfort zone is gone, and big life decisions are being made. It is often so sad to see people who are in the beginning stages of adulthood and in their prime to have a sudden onset of mental illness. Luckily, if treated aggressively, mental illness won't be as impairing as one believes, and many live to complete their goals and aspirations.

If you are suspecting you or your loved one of potentially having a mental illness, it is necessary to be checked by a mental health professional. The presentation of mental illness is not black and white or so clear cut. The onset of mental illness can be very sudden, almost overnight. You see a child happy and lively one day; the next day, they are paranoid and talking to people you don't see. Onset can also be gradual, which provides a confusing time for both the person experiencing it and those around them. Illnesses, like schizophrenia, may creep up with the starting of some suspicion that people at work are talking behind your back. Months later, you may start to feel that they are meeting at your Starbucks to gather more information about you and to talk more. In all, though, you are still functioning, working, and socializing with others. Over the course of more months, you begin to feel that they have put recording software on your computer to further frame you in a job crime you are not a part of. Then finally, you start to confront these people, maybe yell at them, or tell your family who looks at you in shock. This slow, insidious onset can be very deceptive to those around the person who is experiencing this. Many hours and days may be spent with your loved one, trying to investigate these suspicions or talking to lawyers, or even having them change jobs only to find out the same thoughts are now occurring at the new job. It's important to recognize that both these onsets can occur, so don't "write off" what you are observing and fail to get your loved one seen by a mental health professional.

Identifying Mental Illnesses

In the next chapters, you will see the different mental illnesses, the signs and symptoms, tips, and wisdom regarding understanding the mental illness, and the "through their eyes" perspective. Of course, we will not cover the full 287 diagnoses in the DSM-5, but we will cover the major diagnoses seen most prevalently as well as those with the most intensive treatment. The description and information in these sections are never a replacement for a professional mental health clinician. Everyone is different, and many mental illnesses overlap. The purpose and intent is to provide wisdom on each mental illness so that you may recognize when to seek treatment for either yourself or your loved one. In this book, we will focus mostly on the biological understanding of mental illness. There are multitude of approaches to mental health, but I chose biological for two reasons: it is my training, and it is the modality that insurances and the mental health system as a whole uses, thus your most readily available treatment options are based on the biological approach

3

MOOD DISORDERS

Mood disorders are disruptions in every day, productive mood. The mood is seen as temporary states, and we can all agree to this. In general, I may be ornery in the morning, but then happy when I get to work because I learned there was free lunch today, followed by irritability in the afternoon knowing I have to go to the gym and exercise when I'm tired. Mood is on a spectrum, and there is an optimal range in mood that helps us experience our emotions but also keeps us functioning. It's appropriate to be sad when something bad happens and to be happy and excited when something good happens. When the mood goes outside this range, impairment can start to happen, and that's where mood disorders live.

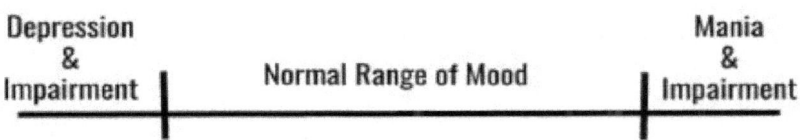

Figure 2.1 The Spectrum of Mood

Mood disorders range from anxiety to depression to bipolar, which then have their subcategory diagnoses such as panic disorder (anxiety) or major depressive disorder (depression). Mood disorders have episodic states, where the person may have a depressive "episode" that last more than two weeks, but then has times of mood stability. This will be different from later discussed diagnoses such as schizophrenia and personality disorders. We will get started with the different disorders and their characteristics.

Depressive Disorders

Major Depressive Disorder

Prevalence: 7% of the population

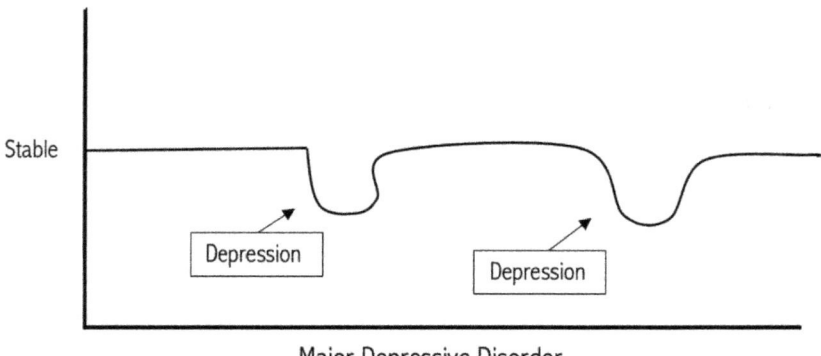

Major Depressive Disorder

Figure 2.2 Major Depressive Disorder has elements of a stable mood with distinct episodes of depression

Signs and Symptoms

- Depressed mood including feelings of emptiness, hopelessness, helplessness
- Lack of pleasure in activities once providing pleasure
- Weight gain or weight loss
- Energy is agitated or maybe retarded (slow to think, slow to move)
- Fatigue or low energy
- Feelings of being worthless or having severe guilt and shame
- Ability to think is disturbed, often with difficulty concentrating or making decisions
- Suicidal thoughts that may be impulsive or well-planned

Brain Function

There is a tremendous amount of research on depression, which has won the award for being the biggest disability in the world, according to the World Health Organization (WHO). There is a consensus that certain chemicals are at play in major depressive disorder. These include the chemical that gives you a sense of well-being (serotonin), a sense of pleasure and motivation (dopamine), and the ability to concentrate and think clearly (norepinephrine). When these chemicals become dysregulated, the body will depress and find little motivation to do much of anything. Serotonin especially is key in depression as its lowering makes us depressed but also makes us anxious and impulsive. You will see later that antidepressant medications often treat anxiety as well. For this reason, when the brain is depressed, the decision making and rational center of the brain (prefrontal cortex) becomes foggy and poor. Unfortunately, when the brain becomes depressed, what follows is irrationality and impulsiveness. This is a detrimental recipe for events like suicide as the person can have great difficulty seeing a future where life is better and becomes a product of intrusive thoughts that are very difficult to control.

Through Their Eyes

Major depressive disorder to the sufferer is a very profound event. To reach a low and have a view of the world that nothing is worthwhile is frightening and also foreign. To someone with major depression, the lens into the future is like looking into the fog — you can't see anything, and it seems that there is really nothing beyond it. Andrew Solomon, a sufferer of depression, wrote a highly acclaimed book on depression, *The Noonday Demon: An Atlas of Depression*, along with doing a TED Talk on depression. Andrew's summation of depression is very powerful and captures the essence of depression — "the opposite of depression is vitality." Vitality is the essence that gives us a reason, and energy to move forward, the liveliness of working toward your goals. For someone that is depressed, this is completely shattered, and the pieces seem insurmountable even to pick up and try to figure out how to put it back together. As a loved one for someone with depression, it's important to recognize that the depressed person will feel alienated and isolated.

Isolation is the general pull of depression due to feelings of not being understood and having the energy to be around others. This further potentiates more depression. Socializing, even with a best friend of the person, can do wonders for those in depression. Being validated for being depressed is also crucial and can help to create a feeling that people understand and care. Thoughts of suicide may be given in signs as a means to tell the person that this is very serious, and I need help to survive it. Others may be so far along the path of depression that they feel there isn't even a point to try and inform others of a planned demise. They will tend to shroud in secrecy and if they do complete suicide, it will be tragic and absolutely shocking to loved ones who really had no chance of knowing the suffering was occurring. The depressed person generally sees a big barrier wall to a lot of suggestions that are made by loved ones. This may include treatment options, or simple "a walk in the park is going to help you." To them, the aspect of hope and imagination that they may be better is completely destroyed and leads to a failure of positive expectations. Intrusive thoughts are common for depressed persons. They are generally very negative, tend to focus on how "awful" or "useless" they are. These intrusive thoughts are very hard to stop, and after some time, the person not only believes it but becomes resistant to others' views of them, which may be positive. People with depression tend to have a high internal locus of control, meaning that they tend to take all problems and issues personally and attributed to all their actions; there is no chance of the environment being out of their control or that there is unpredictability that is not controllable. All decisions and outcomes are solely the faults of the person who is depressed.

Treatment: Psychotherapy, Anti-Depressant, Anti-Anxiety, Anti-psychotics

Similar Disorders: Bipolar Disorder, Cyclothymia, Dysthymia

Bipolar Disorders

Bipolar 1 Disorder and Bipolar 2 Disorder

Prevalence: 1-2% of the general population

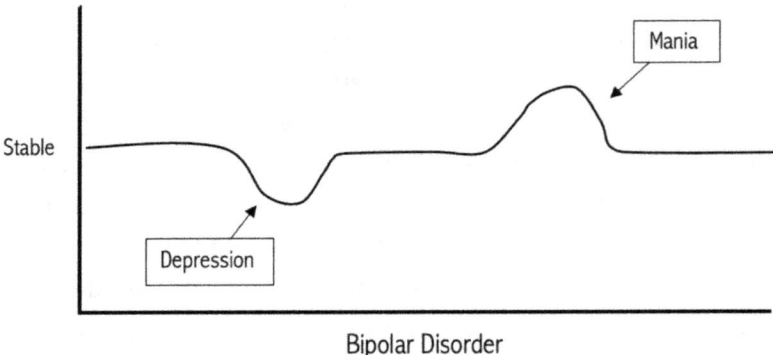

Figure 2.3 Bipolar Disorder has distinct episodes of depression, distinct episodes of mania, and distinct episodes of stability

Signs and Symptoms

Bipolar disorder is broken into two mood states: depression and mania. Further, bipolar disorder has two types: 1 and 2.

Bipolar 1 Disorder

Bipolar 1 Disorder is generally seen as having both major depressive episodes and also full mania episodes. Depending on the person, some people with bipolar 1 disorder may be more prone to having lots of manic episode with very few depressive episodes. The truth can happen in the other direction, where the person experiences more depressive episodes than manic episodes. We see bipolar 1 disorder as having full strength or intense mania episodes compared to bipolar 2 disorder, where the manic episodes are less intense, often never requiring hospitalization. Mania can present with psychotic symptoms (delusions and hallucinations) as well as during depressive episodes.

Depression Episodes	**Mania Episodes**
• Low, depressed mood	• High distractibility
• Poor sleep (too much/too little)	• Rapid speech and Hyperverbal
• Poor eating (too much/too little)	• Racing thoughts
• Poor energy	• Grandiosity (superiority)
• Body either slows down or agitates	• Endless energy
• No pleasure in things once pleasurable	• Little to no sleep without lethargy
• Low motivation	• Agitation
• Suicidal thoughts	• Impulsive (drugs, sex, gambling)
	• Euphoria ("everything is wonderful")
	• Highly social and inappropriate

Table 2.1: Bipolar Disorder Signs and Symptoms

Bipolar 2 Disorder

Bipolar 2 disorder has all the features of bipolar 1 disorder, but the mania is to a lesser intensity (hypomania). People with bipolar 2 disorder tend to have more profound depression and also more frequent episodes of depression than hypomania episodes. You can see that this can be an issue with diagnosis as there are many people with bipolar 2 disorder who were first diagnosed with major depressive disorder. On this same rationale, there are many people with undiagnosed bipolar 2 disorder because they only receive treatment when they are depressed, or the hypomania isn't severe enough to be noticed or considered. Typically, people with bipolar 2 disorder will have episodes of hypomania that involve being highly productive, maybe write a 40-page paper in a day and find themselves to be incredibly creative. Lack of sleep with high energy tends to last only 2-4 days compared to bipolar

1 disorder, which tends to be over seven days. Hypomania does not have a psychotic component and is never intense enough to be hospitalized for. If a person is hospitalized with bipolar 2 disorder and is in their mania state, they automatically upgrade to bipolar 1 disorder due to impairment from the mania. Hypomania can be very useful. It can be channeled to create many innovative ideas. Many entrepreneurs and inventors have bipolar 2 disorder. It gives them that edge and energy to create new innovations. Typically, depression is the main focus of bipolar 2 disorder, as it can be very severe. Hypomania includes all the symptoms of mania in Table 2.1, but to a lesser intensity and typically only involves having 1-3 of the symptoms.

Brain Function

Bipolar disorder involves many areas of the brain and is complicated by the dysregulation of many brain chemicals. To simplify, the brain chemical *dopamine* has a critical role in mania episodes. Dopamine is that brain chemical that rewards you and makes you motivated when something great happens. You can see that when you are manic, dopamine is flooding the brain, everything is great and feels good. Your thoughts have endless energy and potential, so you are ultra-motivated to pursue all of them. Too much dopamine is indicated for mania, but also too much dopamine can cause psychosis, and this is why upwards of 60% of mania episodes have psychotic features. Another brain chemical *glutamate* is increased in the mania episode. Glutamate is an excitatory chemical, fueling the rapid brain fire and making it run on higher energy. This explains the high energy, decreased need for sleep and rapid speech and thought. There also are dysregulations in the brain structures, especially between the prefrontal cortex (decision making and impulse control) and the limbic system (flight, fight, fear, lust). In the depressive episode, the same brain chemicals that are seen in depressive disorders are involved. These include the brain chemicals *serotonin, dopamine,* and *norepinephrine.* These brain chemicals are typically lower when in the depressive stage. There is still much research and clarity needed for understanding the biological principles of bipolar disorder.

Through Their Eyes

The world of bipolar disorder is intriguing. Think of a high where you almost feel angelic, perfected, and so creative that everything you do is amazing and world-renowned only to be met with deep sustaining depression, typically with lots of shame and guilt. The ideas that seemed harmless and "fun" at the time (in mania) may be seen now as "ruining my life." Indeed, anyone with bipolar disorder understands the tribulations faced simply from this brain illness. Having to ask for forgiveness for behaviors done while manic, having to explain how sorry you are for cheating on your significant other, or having to go to a bankruptcy lawyer because you were caught at work high or simply lost your job due to aggressively yelling at your boss. The events are limitless and scary, yet medications don't ever seem like a good answer to all this. Why? Because they can "make you feel dull" or "not me," which is very important to anybody. Typically, in depression and anxiety, the sufferer will do pretty much anything to rid of it. In bipolar disorder, there is always this element of wanting to keep the illness in anticipation of that amazing experience called mania. Mania experiences tell the person that everything is amazing but that everything from now on will be amazing; it's an illusion the illness performs. Simply stated, those who try telling the person that they need to stop these behaviors or that something is wrong clearly does not understand how "great" the person is, which means they don't understand; thus, their opinion of the person is rendered powerless.

Treatment: Psychotherapy, Anti-Depressant, Anti-Anxiety, Anti-psychotics, Mood Stabilizers

Similar Disorders: Borderline personality disorder, ADHD, PTSD

Anxiety Disorders

Panic Disorder

Prevalence: 2-3% of the population

Signs and Symptoms

- Abrupt, sudden, and typically unexpected panic lasting minutes
- Palpitations (heart pounding), high heart rate
- Intense sweating
- Shaking or trembling
- Shortness of breath and difficulty in breathing often felt like smothering
- Choking sensations
- Chest pain likened to a heart attack
- Abdominal distress (nausea, vomiting)
- Lightheadedness
- Chills or extreme heat sensation
- Numbness and tingling sensations
- Fear of going "crazy" (losing control)
- Extreme fear that you may die due to these symptoms

  *At times, panic attacks can lead to dissociation (a feeling that you are not in reality or being detached from yourself)

Brain Function

Panic disorder is incredibly uncomfortable due to the extreme symptoms experienced during a panic attack. Like depression, research shows a dysregulation in the brain chemical serotonin in panic disorder. This leads to impulsivity and anxiety that can lead to extreme attacks of panic. In panic disorder, the fear center of the brain (limbic system) is running amuck and is hypersensitive. It is easily triggered, and when it is activated, it is very hard to stop it. The hypersensitivity of the fear center of the brain leads to unpredictable panic attacks, which seem to come out of nowhere. When panic occurs, the fear center activates the sympathetic nervous system, which is your fight or flight system. If there is not a matching environmental cause to the reaction of the sympathetic nervous system, the body is incredibly uncomfortable and leads to general confusion for the victim. The body reaction is similar to getting shot by a gun but without actually being shot by a gun.

Through Their Eyes

For those who experience panic attacks, going outside or to any place where they feel uncomfortable may be avoided. This is called agoraphobia, which is a fear that one may lose control or become disabled without the ability to escape to a safe place. This is due to the unpredictability as the sufferer cannot usually identify why and how these attacks are happening. The fear can be so profound that the person is almost thrown in a state of delirium where everything around them is a threat and that is to be absolutely avoided. To the sufferer, there is intense panic and discomfort followed by an exhaustion period where one may sleep for a few hours, only to wake up in a panic and go through the cycle again. People tend to suffer higher frequency of panic attacks either in the morning or the nighttime. For the morning, it may be when the person wakes up and is suddenly hit with the thought that they are back in reality where "things are not okay" and hit suddenly with a massive sense of dread. At times, nighttime will have a sudden succession of panic attacks, perhaps due to exhaustion from the day and the body unable to cope with any more stress. The sufferer may avoid any situation they deem to be a trigger for panic. This can include work, school, or even going to a grocery store or calling on the phone. There may be thoughts of suicide due to the perception that the panic attacks will never end, and one cannot fathom going through life with feeling completely out of control.

Treatment: Psychotherapy, Anti-Depressant, Anti-Anxiety

Similar Disorders: Specific phobia, Stimulant abuse, Alcohol withdrawal, Post Traumatic Stress Disorder

* If you or a loved one is experiencing a suspected panic attack and it is the first time, always go to the emergency department or call 911. There is a reason why panic attacks mimic symptoms of other medical emergencies. It would be disastrous to assume a panic attack when it may be an underlying medical emergency.

Generalized Anxiety Disorder (GAD)

Prevalence: 3-8% of the population

Signs and Symptoms

- Excessive worry and apprehension lasting more than six months
- Difficulty to stop worrying
- Restlessness
- Easily fatigued
- Difficulty concentrating or making decisions
- Irritability
- Tension of muscles (feeling "wound up")
- Insomnia or poor sleep quality

Brain Function

Certain amounts of anxiety can be motivating and gives a person a sense that what is causing is anxiety is important. When these levels reach a level that is seen in generalized anxiety disorder, the person is left with a sense of constant worrying, snappiness, and inability to complete tasks due to the anxiety. Research demonstrates that the brain chemical serotonin is once again positioned as the main chemical involved with a generalized anxiety disorder. Another brain chemical, known as GABA, may also be dysregulated. GABA is a brain chemical that helps us feel calm and relaxed. Interestingly enough, alcohol and benzodiazepines (Ativan, Xanax, Valium) raise GABA which is what makes us feel calm and relaxed. There also seems to be evidence that the fear center of the brain (limbic system) is hypersensitive in people who have a generalized anxiety disorder.

Through Their Eyes

People with generalized anxiety disorder tend to have a worry that is out of proportion to the actual thing they are worried about. They may worry and have high anxiety about doing a school assignment because they may "fail" the class if they don't do an absolutely good job. This can lead to procrastination or avoiding the task at hand. The anxiety is experienced across many different aspects of their life. It can be related to their job and doing well at it, to anxiety about the laundry not being done, to worry that a significant other who hasn't come home yet and they are 10 minutes later than when they typically arrive. This can lead to irritability, conflict with others over the anxiety felt, and emotional lability, where their emotions may become dysregulated when the worrying becomes too much (crying, yelling). To people with generalized anxiety disorder, being told "don't worry about it" is not going to work. They have great difficulty stopping the worrying, and often when told to "snap out of it," they will get even more anxiety because they now have new stress to worry about, which is appeasing others. People with generalized anxiety disorder tend to think in black and white — it can either be this or that — and generally have a failure of seeing the grey in events. A term called "catastrophizing" is often experienced by people with generalized anxiety disorder where they face a stressor and expect the worst.

An example is "my husband isn't home yet, and it's been 15 minutes past his normal arrival time, this means he doesn't care and is seeing another person and is planning on leaving me". To those with generalized anxiety disorder, they may see this type of thinking as "preparing for the worst" but also have difficulty recognizing how impairing this can be and how detrimental it can be to those around them. When a generalized anxiety disorder is severe, most can have depression due to their perception that they are "defective" and due to the break down in their relationships. It is typically at this stage that they may be open to treatment with the suggestion coming from a loved one.

Treatment: Psychotherapy, Anti-Depressant, Anti-Anxiety

Similar Disorders: Post Traumatic Stress Disorder, Obsessive Compulsive Disorder, Stimulant Abuse

Obsessive Compulsive Disorder (OCD)

Prevalence: 1-2% of the population

Signs and Symptoms

- Obsessive Thoughts: recurrent, intrusive, disturbing, unwanted and causes distress
- These obsessions are incredibly difficult to control
- Compulsive Behaviors: driven actions in response to obsessive thoughts that are rigid in their execution
- These compulsive behaviors are seen to relieve the distressing obsessive thoughts
- These thoughts and behaviors are very time consuming, often stopping the person in their tracks until the behaviors are completed

Brain Function

Research generally points to the brain chemical serotonin as the main chemical that is dysregulated in OCD. There is some evidence that certain brain structures may have some abnormalities in OCD, mostly with the part of the brain that deals with impulse control and decision making (prefrontal cortex) and the part of the brain that deals with learning, emotion, and thinking (basal ganglia).

Through Their Eyes

Most people who have OCD are completely aware that they are suffering from OCD. For them, it's a challenge to consider treatment because the obsessions and compulsions are so ingrained and so strong that there doesn't seem to be any hope of it ever getting better. People with OCD do not do well when a person tells them to stop their compulsions. This tends to intensify the compulsions, which can lead to more discomfort. The person with OCD knows that the compulsions are absurd and generally fight and resist the obsessive thoughts. It should be noted that people with OCD have been doing their best to control it from the beginning. The repeated failures of not being able to control the obsessions and compulsions can lead to depression and a profound sense of hopeless.

Treatment: Psychotherapy, Anti-Depressant

Similar Disorders: Specific phobias, Eating disorders, Substance abuse, Psychotic disorders

Social Anxiety Disorder

Prevalence: 7%, more in females

Signs and Symptoms

- Fear or apprehension in social settings where the person feels that they will be ridiculed or scrutinized. This includes talking, being observed, or performing (speech)
- Fear that the way they act will lead to humiliation and rejection or both
- Due to this fear, there is the avoidance of social encounters where the fear may occur
- Fear is out of proportion to the actual threat, is lasting over six months, and is impairing in functioning

Brain Function

Social Anxiety Disorder tends to have similar brain structural abnormalities as other anxiety disorders. It should be noted that social anxiety has a very large learned behavior component, meaning that social anxiety is more about learning that social situations are detrimental and then blowing the negative outcomes out of proportion. Nonetheless, there is evidence that the brain's fear center is hypersensitive in social anxiety disorder. It is thought that the brain chemical serotonin (feel-good brain chemical) is involved and, when too low, makes the brain's fear center more sensitive to the environment.

Through Their Eyes

Social anxiety is a constant dread feeling that leads the person to have intense and intrusive thoughts that everything will go wrong or that they will be made fun of. This hypersensitivity leads to irrational thoughts to do anything to "get out of" the situation. To someone socially anxious, missing a wedding, or failing a class to avoid a speech is perfectly feasible to feel better. For them, they may be called "shy," but this is an intense feeling of fear that is very uncontrollable. I have, in my practice, seen people with social anxiety switch careers completely to accommodate their social anxiety. "Getting better" does not seem obtainable and many times, they feel extreme shame and low self-esteem that they cannot "do what others can."

Treatment: Psychotherapy, Anti-Depressant, Anti-Anxiety

Similar Disorders: Schizoid personality disorder, Generalized anxiety disorder, Post traumatic stress disorder

Specific Phobias

Prevalence: 7-9%

Signs and Symptoms

- Intense fear of a specific object or situation (trigger)
- Includes snakes, spiders, flying, heights, injections, others
- This trigger sparks intense fear immediately
- Due to the fear, avoidance is key
- It is impairing in their everyday life and obligations

Brain Function

Like social phobia disorder, specific phobias are generally a learned behavior but typically with the person unable to recall a certain event. Yet, like social phobia, there is evidence of a hypersensitive fear center (limbic). The brain chemical involved with well-being (serotonin) is believed to be involved. Specific phobias tend to occur with other anxiety disorders, such as generalized anxiety disorder and panic disorder.

Through Their Eyes

Specific phobias may not be as daunting in everyday life like other mental disorders, but to those who have specific phobias, the phobia is a source of extreme shame and can lead to very low self-esteem. Thoughts of being "a loser" or "defective" may be common in those with specific phobias as they see others who can engage seemingly effortlessly with the feared trigger. Take flying. A person with specific phobia to flying will feel very alienated because they see so many people who fly without issue. To the person suffering from specific phobia, being asked why they are fearful of the trigger is often very vulnerable and will tend to leave the person stunned and feeling like they have been "caught" being "defective."

Treatment: Psychotherapy, Anti-Depressant, Anti-Anxiety

Similar Disorders: Panic disorder, social anxiety disorder, PTSD

4

PSYCHOSIS DISORDERS

"People who are different are constantly dealing with families who don't understand them"
-Andrew Solomon

Psychosis is challenging for both the person experiencing it and for those who are trying to help the person. It distorts reality rendering the person with difficulty telling what is real and what is not. Psychosis in and by itself can be caused by many factors, including certain mental illnesses, dementia, infections, sleep deprivation, certain medications, and abused substances (especially stimulants like methamphetamine). Psychosis, in the psychiatric field, has two components: hallucinations and delusions. We will also discuss the issue of "insight," which is how the person can recognize that they are not well.

Unfortunately, psychosis can be difficult to treat because so much of the time, the person afflicted has difficulty seeing that they need treatment. Add to this that they are adults that have full autonomy over their health decisions, and you have a recipe for further deterioration. In many ways, psychotic episodes can be seen like heart attacks: the more you have them, the worse and harder it is to treat. In modern medicine, if a person has a heart attack, they are treated very aggressively to prevent another heart attack that can kill precious heart tissue. Psychosis wreaks havoc on the brain, yet modern psychiatry doesn't treat psychotic episodes like a "heart attack," and many times, families or loved ones simply have no clue (due to poor teaching from clinicians) that each psychotic episode is very detrimental to the brain. There is good evidence that after each psychotic episode, the brain is typically harder to treat, and their symptoms become worse (increasing the baseline in clinical terms).

An example is a lifelong homeless man with schizophrenia. His life has been in and out of the hospitals, off then on medications, and having a lovely jail stay every once and awhile. Full-blown treatment of antipsychotics (the latest and greatest), as well as a whole array of other psychiatric cocktails and, yet, the person may only be slightly better. You will then hear clinicians say, "this is their baseline," meaning that their baseline (normal) is that of a chronically psychotic state. The human brain can only take so much chemical toxicity and damage. In many ways, these are brains that are race cars but without the oil being changed or running out of gas frequently, or not getting general maintenance. It, unfortunately, takes its tragic toll on the person along with nature's cruel trick of making the mind not able to recognize that there is an illness and suffering from it.

Hallucinations

Hallucinations include any of the five senses becoming haywire. By far, the most common type of hallucination is auditory. Auditory hallucinations vary dramatically from background "white noise" to actual people with names and saying specifics to the person suffering. Visual hallucinations are the next most common type of hallucination. Once again, these can vary from specks of light in the corner of the eyes to full-blown people and scenery in front of the person suffering. The next type of hallucinations involves touch, taste, and smell. Although these are rarer, they certainly do occur. In my practice, I had a patient with severe schizophrenia who constantly had feelings that people were spitting on him. He would subsequently spit at random people leading to an interesting day being his nurse.

Delusions

Delusions are incredibly complex by their nature because the person believes that the delusions are true. To the person, it is as real as you waking up this morning or using the restroom. They are false and fixated and do not make sense with evidence or with the general perspective of reality. Common delusions include

- **Grandiose:** These include thoughts of being greater than others or maybe even supernatural. Common thoughts include having mind-reading capabilities or believing they know when Jesus will come back.
- **Persecutory:** These delusions include thoughts that people are trying to kill them or hurt them. Sometimes the theme may be a "sacrifice" to "save others." Other times, it may be that they are being poisoned, drugged, conspired against, or a grand plan to destroy their livelihood. You can see that this type of delusion is similar to paranoia
- **Paranoid:** This can include thoughts that the government is after the person or maybe that the inheritance is secretly being switched to the other sibling. Paranoid delusions are very common, and they can range greatly. Some are so subtle that you do wonder if what the person is stating is actually happening, while other times, it is blatant as blatant can be. Around 2010, I had a long-standing patient who I treated that believed that the government was after him because his "girlfriend" was named "Isis," which happened to be all over the news during the Syrian Civil War. His proclamation to me was to let me know that he needed a bus ticket to the Los Angeles Federal Court to "declare war on the United States" because the U.S. was trying to kill his girlfriend, "Isis."
- **Somatic:** these delusions are involved with physical conditions, either sensation or function. Such a delusion may be that "there is a tumor

in my stomach," yet, all tests state that there is no tumor. Others may include thoughts that their body is infested with worms or maggots
- **Erotomania:** these delusions tend to be on the rare side but involve false ideas that certain people are infatuated or in love with the person. Such delusions lead to severe issues with romantic relationships, for both the sufferer's relationship and the person accused relationship
- **Idea of Reference:** these delusions are very common and often the stem of many jokes, unfortunately. These delusions involve aspects of telepathy, the ability to read minds, or that their mind is being read. Sometimes it's the government that puts a "chip" in them and is monitoring them. Another common thread is that the television is telling them secret messages or that they are receiving messages through music
- **Hyper-Religious:** these delusions involve themes of religion, mostly related to the religion the person is affiliated with. They may focus on being "the chosen one" or seeing "God" in all sorts of different mediums, such as the wall or by the way someone talks. The mind is heavily preoccupied with these themes to the point of impairment and relationship deterioration

Delusions and how they occur is always an intriguing topic in the world of mental health. Normally, our brains pick up on events or objects around us and make sense of our environment. When in tune, our brain will focus on the necessary stimuli (objects) and turn off the other stimuli that aren't necessary. This is done through a brain chemical called dopamine. Dopamine is a fascinating brain chemical and is seen in all areas of mental health, from depression and addiction to schizophrenia and psychosis. Dopamine is mostly known for its role in our reward center. When I eat that snickers bar I love, I get a blast of dopamine that not only feels good but motivates me to seek more of it out (Can someone say addiction?). Dopamine reinforces behaviors and types of stimuli we pay attention to. This is why it's easier to watch an action film and get excited (from dopamine) than say reading a technical book (less dopamine). One of the theories of psychosis is that dopamine is very high in the brain. Antipsychotics, which we'll get to in a later chapter, work primarily by lowering dopamine, which helps alleviate delusions and hallucinations.

We know that dopamine is what rewards us when our body likes something, but it is also known to aid in focusing, concentration, and ability to regulate stimuli. Let me explain by example. Right now, I'm sitting at a coffee shop typing this world-famous book that you are reading now. My focus is on the thoughts in my head regarding the book, focusing on my screen, typing correctly and noticing my type of errors. Dopamine is helping guide me by giving little bits of dopamine to each one of these tasks. It is not giving me dopamine bits for also listening to all the people around me or the sounds of the coffee machine, or the cars passing by, or the sun reflecting off of a window, or the newspapers being stacked, and more. If it did do this, I would be completely overwhelmed and not able to delegate my attention and understanding of my environment very well. Luckily, my brain is regulating dopamine to be able to pick up on the right stimuli, in the right amount, and at the right times.

In psychosis, there is access to dopamine in the brain. This leads the brain to start making everything noticeable (called salience). Could you imagine if I was picking up on all those other stimuli while typing as if they are just as important to be in my focus as the writing of this book? The excess dopamine overwhelms the brain with picking up stimuli, and that makes it difficult to discern what is the reality and what is not. My brain is saying that the newspapers are stacked in a certain order, which my brain is telling me has a tremendous purpose right now. This is something that needs to be focused on and understood because the importance meter is very high right now. It must have meaning. This is where the brain gets in trouble with altered realities. Suddenly, our pattern-seeking brain is formulating all sorts of patterns based on a faulty system. These are many false alarms but are not discernable.

Figure 2.4 Reality viewed as a TV screen, playing the one channel, for the normal brain

You will see people who are experiencing psychosis being what we call "internally preoccupied". This is seen when the person has that 1000 yard stare, and they are not in tune with their surroundings. They are stuck in their brains with all these increased stimuli. You typically have to start to engage them, and then they will focus on the conversation, but you'll see that this takes energy and is very difficult to maintain. An example that I have heard before explains this idea very well. For the regulated person, there is one "TV screen" we focus on during the day, it is a reality, and our brains are regulating dopamine to make sure we pick up on the right objects in the environment and wash out the other stuff. For the person in psychosis, they have multiple "TV screens" going all at one time, each with different shows, and the brain is saying all these are important and true. When we are talking to a person with psychosis, and when they are presented with these delusions, they are simply telling you about the other "TV screen with a different episode." Add hallucinations that are visual or auditory telling you that this "TV screen" is more important or more serious or "the truth," and you can begin to fathom the overwhelming nature of psychosis.

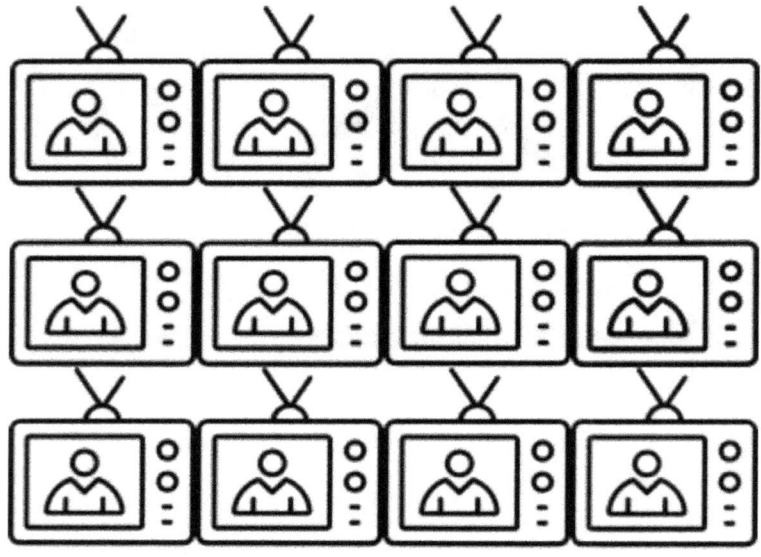

Figure 2.5 Through the Psychotic Brain – multiple realities appear due to "picking" up on an array of patterns.

You can see how sometimes psychosis can bring on disorganized speech. I may ask a person with schizophrenia, "how many siblings do you have?" and they may respond verbatim with varying responses such as: "100,000, but not spiritual.....three and a half brothers....half, because a hand was cut off....he ran to Saudi Arabia....talking to trees." This was an actual response to an assessment I was performing. It may be that he perceives these multiple screens. Maybe one is of a crowd of 100,000 people at a concert coming together with another screen of Saudi Arabia and the punishment of stealing by cutting off the hand of the thief with another screen of seeing a person talking to a tree because he appreciates nature. Maybe he does have three brothers and a half brother but mixed in with the other realities, and the result is a garbled mash of realities (screens). Can you imagine how frustrating it must be to have to communicate to others when your brain is tricking you like this?

Psychosis is most often seen in the following disorders: schizophrenia, schizoaffective, bipolar, and major depression

Insight

Insight is the ability of the person to recognize that there is something wrong or having a complete unawareness (*anosognosia*). Poor to no insight is incredibly common in psychosis and also in bipolar disorder, especially in the mania phase. Having little to no insight is very detrimental to the health of the person suffering and to those around them as they must contend to a world that can wreak havoc and yet have no ability to convince the person that they are not well. It is estimated that around 50% of those with psychosis and bipolar or both conditions will experience little to no insight.

The hardest cases that I have experienced was with a person not having any idea that they are not well. They may sabotage relationships, fight (sometimes physically) with their loved ones, give all their assets away, stop their medications, go on an impromptu trip far away, or quit their job. The complete unawareness for years was seen as an extreme form of "denialism" to protect the integrity of the person who was doing all these detrimental behaviors. We in the mental health field have moved on from this notion with the advent of neuroscience. It is widely believed that the areas of the brain that give us our "self" are grossly awry when a person has no insight (typically psychotic or manic). They literally cannot fathom the reality you are telling them. It is incredibly real to them despite everyone they know telling them it's the complete opposite. Because of the masses going against the person, the person with little to no insight will see them as an "enemy" or as a person who "doesn't get it," which can lead to some of the drastic behaviors mentioned above. I have unfortunately seen so many family and social networks destroyed over the symptom of little to no insight. To repeat these episodes that can cause so much havoc, many who care for the person can only take so much.

I highly recommend reading the book, *I am not sick, I don't need help*, by Dr. Xavier Amador, who is a leader in research on insight and mental illness. His book is highly acclaimed and a very popular resource for family and friends who are in the midst of a loved one who has little to no insight. His well-known *LEAP (Listen, Empathy, Agree, Partner)* technique is internationally acclaimed and contains an evidenced-based intervention for people with little to no insight.

Even with such good resources, the issue of insight will continue to be a tense issue in the future. What do you do if someone is causing so much damage to themselves or others, and they have no clue that they are even doing it? How much should a family endure before making that awful decision to cut ties? How do we hold and force people to take medications when they have no insight? Many of the controversies in the mental health community stem from this issue, from the intimate relationship to the government policy, saying that providers can "conserve" someone due to poor insight. The implications are also the main user of healthcare dollars because of the frequent deterioration of the person, who then will be readmitted, started on medications again, only to stop the medications and repeat the cycle.

Schizophrenia

Prevalence: Around 1% of the population

Signs and Symptoms

Schizophrenia is generally broken into two symptoms categories. Some people with schizophrenia may be more of one type than the other or may have a blend of the two types. Also, schizophrenia lies on a spectrum, meaning that you may have some with schizophrenia who have very light symptoms and are very high functioning (managing own home, employment, engaged in treatment). You may also have some with schizophrenia who have severe symptoms and are, in the classic sense, very disabled.

These two symptoms groups are broken into **Positive symptoms** and **Negative symptoms**

Positive Symptoms	Negative Symptoms
➢ Hallucinations	➢ Flat or Little Emotion
➢ Delusions	➢ Little Social Interest
➢ Disorganized Speech	➢ Lack of Enjoyment Experienced
➢ Inappropriate Affect (laughing at nothing)	➢ Little Motivation Observed
➢ Disorganized Movements	➢ Little Attention Used
	➢ Little Speech Use
	➢ Catatonia (Slow or Frozen Movements)

Table 2.2 Positive and Negative symptoms as seen in Schizophrenia

Positive symptoms are remembered as any symptom that is "added" to what we call "normal" behavior. So, symptoms like hallucinations are in addition to the normal range of human mood and thought. Thus, are delusions too, including paranoia. Negative symptoms are those symptoms that are "deficits" in, again, "normal" behaviors. So, having a face that remains expression-less with little change in emotion is considered to be a deficit in characteristics of the normal range of mood and thought. It can be hard to differentiate these symptoms, but it is important to understand which type your loved one or yourself may be prone to because the treatment can be different. Generally speaking, positive symptoms are easier to treat than negative symptoms, but we will discuss this later.

Brain Function

Schizophrenia is probably one of the most studied mental disorders in the world. Its symptoms and presentation has fascinated many in the world of science. Because of this fascination, science has found sound evidence of how the brain is working in schizophrenia. The first and foremost theory regarding schizophrenia is that there is a high level of the brain chemical, dopamine. As stated before, high levels of this brain chemical have been linked to psychosis (delusions and hallucination) and are the target of antipsychotics. With schizophrenia, there seem to be substantial brain structure differences as well. The part of the brain that helps with what they call "executive functioning" (planning, memory, impulse control, attention, and thought flexibility) appears to have circuitry issues. This part of the brain (prefrontal cortex) is also very important to help us socialize with others. One thing you will see with schizophrenia is typically an inability to connect well with others and tend to disengage in conversations. Because impulse control is inhibited (stopped), they may have reactionary behaviors or also impulsive decision making. There is further research that demonstrates that schizophrenia may be more of a neurological deficit disorder, one that may arise before full-blown schizophrenia. These impairments before schizophrenia can be difficulty in social situations, thinking and attention issues, and maybe even motor or movement skills. Genetics plays a very big role in schizophrenia. If one parent has schizophrenia, there is a 13% chance of passing this on, and if both parents have schizophrenia, then that chance rises to 50%. Please note that there is further research that supports that it doesn't necessarily have to be parents with schizophrenia that increases risk, but can be other mental illness, especially with psychosis involved (bipolar or depression).

Through Their Eyes

When one is experiencing schizophrenia, anything is possible. The shear distortions in reality allow for complex and odd patterns of thought that can transcend any evidential or experiential experiences by most people. Having your senses constantly tricking you while having thoughts that are disorganized and hard to piece together is incredibly frustrating and isolating to anyone with schizophrenia. Often, being a loner and away from people is the only peaceful way of being, this includes being around others with schizophrenia, where typically people with similar disorders benefit from learning from each other. In schizophrenia, natural consequences do not make sense and can spur up at any time, which leaves the person in a world of unpredictability and fear. Paranoia can arise out of the fact that people can be unpredictable and "after" you when really, many times, these are natural consequences of behaviors (being kicked out of school for "preaching" about mass murders, etc.). Having little insight also creates a world that is ultra-confusing. Imagine going to your workplace of 15 years, and out of nowhere, your supervisor comes up and states to you that you cannot come back to work because you have left work early for multiple days and stole food that you deemed to be poisoned. Oh, and if you don't leave right now, the police will be called. Even though these behaviors occurred, to the person, this would catch them off guard and would have a complete inability to see the connection.

Betrayal is a very common emotion experienced by people with schizophrenia or any type of psychosis. Why? Well, because many times they WILL have the police called or family discussion about their need to take medications that will "alter their thoughts" as well as being put into the hospital against their will because family stated there were dangerous or disabling behaviors occurred. In a schizophrenia world where what you think is true and has intense meaning, the thought of your closest loved ones trying to go against that is truly devastating and betraying to the person. So many families and loved ones who experience this know EXACTLY what I am writing as they can be verbally and even physically attacked because of this betrayal feeling that can occur when the person has become very symptomatic and requires treatment. For the family and loved ones, the challenge and difficulty of taking this rage while no logical explanations can pierce the shield of delusions or little insight create absolute havoc on relationships, unfortunately leading to very drastic changes in the family and loved ones' dynamics.

Treatment: Psychotherapy, Antipsychotics

Similar Disorders: Schizoaffective Disorder, Bipolar with psychotic features, Major Depressive Disorder with psychotic features, Substance-induced psychosis

Schizoaffective Disorder (Bipolar Type or Depressed Type)

Prevalence: about 1% of the population

Signs and Symptoms

Schizoaffective Disorder is a combination of schizophrenia and a mood disorder (either bipolar or depression). Thus, the schizoaffective disorder will have elements of both schizophrenia and the specific type of mood disorder.

Schizoaffective Disorder, **Depressed Type** will have schizophrenia elements plus depression episodes.

Schizoaffective, **Bipolar Type** will have schizophrenia elements plus depression episodes and mania episodes

Depression Episodes	Mania Episodes
• Low, depressed mood	• High distractibility
• Poor sleep (too much/too little)	• Rapid speech and Hyperverbal
• Poor eating (too much/too little)	• Racing thoughts
• Poor energy	• Grandiosity (superiority)
• Body either slows down or agitates	• Endless energy
• No pleasure in things once pleasurable	• Little to no sleep without lethargy
• Low motivation	• Agitation
• Suicidal thoughts	• Impulsive (drugs, sex, gambling)
	• Euphoria ("everything is wonderful")
	• Highly social and inappropriate

Brain Function

Schizoaffective disorder is a complicated brain illness. In theory, it has elements of both schizophrenia pathology and a mood disorder pathology. Depending on the type of schizoaffective one has, certain brain areas are affected. Both types of schizoaffective will have a psychosis component, which means that the brain chemical dopamine will be involved. Generally, the theory is that too much dopamine in certain areas (mesolimbic or mesocortical) of the brain causes the psychosis we see in schizoaffective disorder. If the schizoaffective is depressed type, this means that there is a depressive component to the brain. This could include too low of the brain chemicals serotonin, dopamine, and norepinephrine in certain areas of the brain. To make things more complicated, schizoaffective disorder with bipolar type will have all of the above but with mania episodes as well. Mania is generally seen to be an increase in the excitatory brain chemical glutamate, as well as increases in dopamine, leading to the classic mania episodes we see.

Through Their Eyes

Like schizophrenia, schizoaffective disorder completely alters the world of the person experiencing it. The distortions in their psychosis are so real and tangible in the same way you know that you can drink water when you are thirsty. Because of their unique perception of the world, it is an incredibly isolating illness, filled with people who don't understand them, fear them, and typically challenge anything they say. Schizoaffective has the added component of a mood disorder, either bipolar or depression. Because of this, this distorted world is met with extreme fluctuations in moods that can be very unbearable. Suicide is a real concern in the life of someone with schizoaffective disorder due to this deadly combination of psychosis and extreme depression or extreme mania. To those with schizoaffective disorder, medications may appear to be a "trick" to change who they are. They may not want medications because it can dull the extremely sought after mania, which feels amazing. Typically, medications will be more of an option when in depressed moods as they are more likely to want to be out of depression. Remember, we (general public) see giving medications to help with their distorted thoughts, but to those with schizoaffective disorder, they see it as you trying to distort their "normal" reality.

Treatment: Psychotherapy, Anti-Depressant, Antipsychotics, Mood Stabilizers

Similar Disorders: Bipolar with psychotic features, Major depressive disorder with psychotic features, schizophrenia

5

PERSONALITY DISORDERS

"Personality is like a charioteer with two headstrong horses, each wanting to go in different directions."
–Martin Luther King, Jr.

A Primer on Personality

One of the most confusing topics is that of personality disorders. We all have a grasp of someone's "personality," but when we start talking about mood disorders versus personality disorders? Well, what do we have here? Don't worry if you have difficulty determining what a personality disorder is compared to a mood disorder. Nursing students and even mental health professionals can have a difficult time grasping the differences, let alone being able to explain it to someone else.

*Mood: the **temporary** or **transient** state of mind or feeling*

*Personality: the combination of **characteristics** or **qualities** that forms a person's distinctive character*

Mood and thought disorders fall right into this definition. They focus on changes and impairing *episodes* of mood or thought dysregulation. Once stabilized or returned to baseline, the person is "back" to their stable self. Notice the temporary nature of this. You may have panic disorder and have panic attacks for two months straight. After some therapy and maybe some medication, your panic attacks subside, and you return to your stable self. You may go into another episode in the future, but the characteristics (personality) of *you* have been relatively the same during both the panic episodes and stable episode.

Personality disorders become a little more complicated. Our personalities are qualities and characteristics of who we are to ourselves and to those who see us. This interaction between our self-concept and the world plays an extensive role in the formation of our personality. In comparison to mood, personality is rigid, long-lasting, and resistant to change. This is typically a very good thing. Having a strong self-concept and interaction with the world provides stability and outlook on life. If our personality were as fluid as our emotions (as it can be in personality disorders), then the world is a threat to you, constantly unstable, untrustworthy, let alone not feeling you can rely on yourself or your qualities. Of course, we have the popular "extroversion" and "introversion" variation of personality that most of us are familiar of. Think of somebody that is extroverted. You see that their *qualities* of extroversion are seen in their interactions with others, their decisions in life, their view of who they are as a person, and what that means in the world. Can depression do these things too? Certainly, but is much more transient and based on how they feel rather than how they operate.

Personality disorders affect how the person sees their world, interacts with their world, and how they interact or believe about themselves. Mood disorders tend to be an old lovely Freudian word *ego-dystonic*, which is a cool way of saying that when you feel depressed or anxious, this is not in line with your *ego* or balanced self; thus you typically know something is wrong and that you are not at your baseline. Personality disorders, on the other hand, are seen to be *ego-syntonic,* meaning that the impairments lie directly with the ego. They see nothing wrong as this is "their self concept baseline," according to them. It's hard to understand others when they tell you that you are doing things that hurt or are detrimental to a relationship if you don't even understand how you are doing any wrong. Because of this, personality disorders are incredibly hard to treat. Not because there isn't treatment but because it's hard to keep people with personality disorders in treatment, let alone getting them in there in the first place. There simply is *nothing* wrong in their minds. The few treatments for personality disorders, I hate to say, have dismal rates of recovery. It's hard to change or use new ways of thinking when you have difficulty seeing what you are doing is even an issue. Personality disorders focus a lot on how the person interacts with others in society. A borderline personality disorder is notorious for emotional instability and fragmented relationships with people. An antisocial personality disorder is notorious for how acts can be done against people without any remorse or empathy. Unfortunately, the numbers don't look good either. Personality disorders are relatively frequent, and we know that many are out there who have not been treated because remember, they don't typically seek any treatment.

Does that mean if you have a personality disorder that there is no hope? Absolutely not. We are continually learning more about personality disorders and finding that they may be more fluid to change than once believed. Therapies, like dialectical behavioral therapy, are offering hope to people with borderline personality disorder (along with other mental illnesses). At times, a person may be diagnosed with a personality disorder only to find out that they have extensive trauma in their background (very common in personality disorders). You start to treat the trauma, and the personality disorder traits start to dissipate. Some personality disorders are more likely than others to seek treatment, like borderline personality disorder or obsessive-compulsive personality disorder (which is different from obsessive-compulsive disorder). Even after reading this, you may still have that *quoi?* about personality disorders, and that's okay. With time, you will start to see the division between personality and mood, and it will become clearer, especially if you or a loved one has a personality disorder.

A Note...

Because of the nature of the mental health system, only certain personality disorders are relatively seen and spoke about. As stated before, most people with personality disorders can be highly functional, sustain a family, sustain a job, and never even face a psychiatrist or the mental health system. On the other hand, some personality disorders tend to be seen at a higher frequency in both the mental health system and the criminal justice system. This is typically what they call the "cluster B" or "Eccentrics" or "Dramatics" class of personality disorders. These include borderline, antisocial, histrionic, and narcissistic personality disorders. For the sake of this book, we will go over all the personality disorders, but give some special attention to the cluster B personality disorders as they are typically mostly seen in the mental health system, as well as highly asked about by families who have a loved one with a cluster B personality disorder.

The Clusters of Personality Disorders - odd, eccentric, and anxious type

Odd

Schizoid

This personality disorder is not frequently seen in the public. People with schizoid personality disorder tend to have a lack of desire to be around people. This includes family and friends and of course, strangers. A dream for a person with schizoid personality disorder would be a world to roam free and have zero other people in it. They simply don't feel a need to attach to or be around others. Not even having sex with another person is of any interest, instead they prefer masturbation or sexual abstinence. People with a schizoid personality disorder may live in a internal fantasy world of their own, which may look like they are not in tune with reality. Not only do they not want to be around people, when speaking to others, they generally have great difficulty expressing themselves. Rather emotionless, the motivation to express or communicate with others is very low, thus missing that "experience" in reflecting with others about feelings and thoughts, which makes it difficult to express. Generally, the treatment for schizoid personality is none as people with schizoid personality disorder rarely seek treatment. They typically do not see any issue or need to get better. If ever open, traditional treatments include cognitive behavioral therapy and psychodynamic therapy.

Schizotypal

Schizotypal personality disorder is a peculiar disorder and is typically not seen very much. I always think of schizotypal being half social anxiety disorder and half schizophrenia. The reason is that people with schizotypal personality tend to have extreme anxiety around people and generally have very poor people skills. Call it hypersensitivity or paranoia; these people feel very uncomfortable in any relationship, from family to significant other. They tend to hold odd beliefs regarding the world and are very prone to paranormal topics. Such odd thoughts can lead to interesting ways of dress or interesting ways of communicating, such as not responding or simply responding off-topic. Magical ways of thinking, believing in mind control, and paranoia can be hallmarks of schizotypal personality disorder. For this reason, most professionals see schizotypal personality disorder on the schizophrenia spectrum.

Once again, treatment is rarely seen in schizotypal personality disorder as such people don't see anything wrong and can be very high functioning, thus never touching the mental health system. If they do, traditional antipsychotics can be used, although traditionally don't have a good effect. If therapy is an option, highly structured group therapy can aid in socialization skills and comfort with others. This, once again is very rarely seen.

Paranoid

There's a paranoid personality disorder? Isn't that just schizophrenia with paranoia? This is a typical question I get from my students when studying personality disorders, and I can see why there is confusion. Paranoid personality disorder differs from schizophrenia in that the paranoia is personality based. Their personality expresses paranoia and mistrust, most of the time, at a low-level stable expression. Schizophrenia tends to wax and wane, tends to have a period when the disease was not there but diagnosed later in life. People with paranoid personality typically never have hallucinations, or negative symptoms (little emotion), or disorganized thoughts that are often seen in schizophrenia. Instead, they can be very high functioning and stable people. These are the people who you may work with and they'll believe every other person is out to get their job, or to get them fired, or maybe watching their every move. These thoughts don't ebb and flow but are persistent in any environment. They may invest in a heavy video security system for their home and monitor it obsessively or question your intentions when you ask if they live in the area or if their child goes to the same school as your child. You can see they are paranoia and extra caution but not to a level where they can't hold a job or support their needs. This is dramatically different from schizophrenia, which can be incredibly disabling.

Eccentric

Antisocial

In the general population, you tend to hear the word "antisocial" to be that you don't want or feel like being around people. For anyone in the mental health field, this word has a far different meaning that is far more critical than just saying you don't like being around people (which is being asocial). An antisocial personality disorder is characterized by the apparent lack of empathy, coldness, and ability to cause harm, violate others' well-being, and deceive. An antisocial personality disorder is a disorder of self-gratification; the endless game of "I win, you lose" mentality in every interaction they have. Colloquially, antisocial personality shares the terms *psychopath* and *sociopath*. These terms are very familiar in the world of movies, pop culture, documentaries and so on. For the most part, there is no scientific distinguishing between the terms psychopath and sociopath. Some in the field will state there are differences such as psychopathy being more "biological" while sociopathy is more "environmental" based. In the end, the diagnosis will be an antisocial personality disorder. People with antisocial personality disorder tend to come from backgrounds where there were no "prosocial" role models, meaning that antisocial traits were introduced early in development. Neglect in early childhood seems to be a factor along with heavy abuse and sadistic abuses. Nonetheless, there are some with an antisocial personality disorder that had loving parents and in a good up bring. Some biological implications have been found, mostly their low pulse rate in comparison to others and their difficulty in seeing the fear in animals and humans.

Many times, people with antisocial personality disorder began showing signs in childhood. Fighting others and tendencies to hurt (even kill animals) can be red flags. Stealing, property destruction without any form of feeling guilt is also a telltale sign. When these patterns are seen when the person is a minor, they are diagnosed with *conduct disorder*, which is sort of like antisocial personality disorder for people under 18. If the person turns 18 and the traits are still there, they upgrade to antisocial personality disorder. Not every child that has conduct disorder will become antisocial; indeed many don't.

As you can imagine, people with antisocial personality disorder end up clashing with the law. While roughly around 3% of the general population has an antisocial personality disorder, out of that percentage, those in jails and prisons is roughly about 25-30%. Indeed, we understand the serial killer, the lifetime spouse abuser, the petty thief criminal searching for excitement, but what may be more disturbing is the amount of antisocial personality disorder seen in white-collar society. In a competition based society like the United States, antisocial traits can take someone very far because of their "I win, you lose" mentality and no remorse for any of their behaviors. People with antisocial personality disorder have an adverse reaction to "boredom" or "normalcy." They are in a constant striving for excitement and boundary-pushing, typically with dangerous acts. Being highly manipulative, they can tend to present with sincere remorse and convince that they have changed, but their behaviors and future actions will show that, indeed, they have not changed.

Unfortunately, treatment has little options and tends to be useless. One of these reasons is because, like other personality disorders, people with an antisocial personality disorder do not see anything wrong with them. Instead, they tend to blame others for their misfortunes. It wasn't because they were caught stealing a car, it was the police's fault for being vigilant and taking them to jail. It's the lawyers, judges, family, and anyone else's fault but theirs. If you can convince or force in most circumstances, someone with an antisocial personality disorder to attend therapy, they will see this as a "challenge" that they must "win." Indeed, therapy can be more dangerous as the person learns what to say in certain circumstances to appear better. Many therapists, counselors, doctors, and nurses have been completely duped by people with antisocial personality at getting better, building insight, increasing their remorse, only to learn later that they were manipulated, and the person just learned how to use the lingo in the right circumstance.

This makes people with antisocial personality disorder very hard to treat and puts them in a seemingly revolving door with conflict, the law, or loved ones.

Borderline

Borderline personality disorder, probably one of the most stigmatized diagnoses out there next to addiction. People with borderline personality disorder get a bad rap, being called "difficult," "selfish," "dramatic," "crazy," "nuts." Why such a bad rap? Mostly because borderline personality disorder focuses heavily on the relationship with other people, which tends to be toxic. People with borderline personality disorder are poorly understood. Their ways of interacting with life is malfunctioned, extremely emotion-driven, and chronically feeling empty. Most people with borderline personality disorder have a traumatic past, especially in childhood. Indeed, when I hear "borderline," I think "trauma." Most statistics point to the number around 70% of those with borderline personality have experienced significant trauma in their backgrounds, whether physical, emotional, sexual or neglect. People with heavy bias may fight you on this argument that trauma and borderline have close commonalities.

I had a well-established psychiatrist before tell me that I was "'duped" by "borderlines" when I presented him this statistic of 70%. His rationale was that many people have traumatized pasts who never become "borderline" and that "borderlines" are just "grown-up brats." Let's put aside the projection of his inadequacy of not being able to have success with people with borderline personality disorder and look at the logic. Many ailments have commonalities or propensity from certain causes, but not always. Look at high blood pressure. A very common medical disease. We know that eating a high salt, and high-fat diet can lead to high blood pressure, and I'm sure there is a high amount of people with high blood pressure that was caused by high salt and poor eating styles, but that doesn't mean that ALL people who eat high salt and poor diets have to get high blood pressure or that all people with high blood pressure got it from ONLY high salt and poor diet. Many people experience traumatic events, and some may come out okay, some develop PTSD, some don't, some develop a borderline personality disorder, some don't. This doesn't negate the fact that the evidence shows that around 70% of those with borderline personality disorder have experienced trauma, which by the way, is more than those who get PTSD from a traumatic event (around 20%). Okay, I'm ending the rant, I promise.

As challenging as having a borderline personality can be, understanding the mind of borderline personality disorder is crucial. In many ways, it's a result of their past. Borderline personality contains the borderline triad with the three main concepts of the disorder. This includes a poor sense of identity, self-harm behaviors (including substance use), and turbulent interpersonal relationships (especially fear of abandonment).

The first of the triad, poor sense of identity, stems from their feeling that they don't have any traits. They tend to focus on the negative aspects of their feelings rather than who they are. Because of this, they seek to find "perfect ideals" in other people to fill this lack of self-identity and to thrive off their perception of the other person's "great qualities". They will adapt many aspects of themselves to fit the mold of this new person who is to fill in all the needs the person has. This person they see as having these great ideals are inflexible distortions in their minds, thus leading to extreme expectations that the other person is to live up to. Once that person fails, which will surely happen, the person with borderline feels a complete loss of all meaningful identity. Not only that, in traditional black and white thinking, the person with the perfect ideals, is now the worst person imaginable, purposely sabotaging the borderline person's well-being and feeling of safety. This is called *splitting* and is a hallmark of borderline personality disorder. They tend to live in a land of heroes and villain, and all people fall into one or the other to always try to fill this void. But how and why does this happen?

When you look at trauma, especially in childhood, any sense of self-control is shattered. Your brain quickly learns that you can be overpowered and be in fear of your life at any moment. Your brain does not want this to happen again, so it resorts to black and white thinking to easily detect fears, bad vs. good, safe vs. dangerous, savior vs. killer, etc. It is a survival mechanism that becomes out of whack. This ingrained learning then is the filter to all of their life, constantly assessing who is "true" and who is "false," as they do not want to be hurt anymore. Trauma also builds an external locus of control, which is how we gauge how much control we have versus how much we don't have. External locus of control focuses on events occurring from external influences that the person is not in control of, while internal locus of control tends to view that events occurring have control internally within the person. External locus of control is pivotal in borderline life. You are not in control during trauma, the fear and terrible feelings you are having are because this external person is doing this to you without any concern over your control, thoughts, emotions, and input. This shift to an external locus of control puts such high reliability on others to feel control and safe. The issue is that this overburdening pressure on other people will almost certainly fail because other humans are just not capable of tending to every need of the person with borderline.

Self-harm and dangerous behaviors are some other hallmarks of the borderline triad. Extreme begets extreme, and people with borderline experience extreme emotions. Especially in the face of depression, feelings of emptiness, and abandonment fear, people with borderline personality are very prone to self-harm behaviors, such as cutting, burning, or hitting hard objects. When you are hurt physically, your brain releases tons of its opiates (pain killers) called endorphins. This "kills" the emotional pain being experienced and at times, can have you completely dissociate from the painful event. This self-invoked pain killer is frequently used in borderline personality disorder, people with trauma/PTSD, and severe depression. Drug and substance abuse are very common and typically not just one substance, but an array of substances to cover all different emotional states. Sometimes a downer like alcohol for anxiety, meth or Adderall when feeling depressed, or maybe a mishmash of substances to obliterate all feelings completely. Sexual promiscuity can be a feature and having many sexual partners is a common feature of borderline personality disorder. Once again, this is to aid in the temporary high of feeling wanted, important, and pleasure-seeking. Unfortunately, with all these acts of harm, the effect is temporary and only leads to the relentless chronic feelings of self-inadequacy, loneliness, and emotional turmoil.

Suicide attempts or "gestures" tend to be common in borderline personality disorder. Roughly around 70% of people with a borderline personality disorder will attempt suicide. Most suicide attempts by people with borderline personality are not due to them wanting to necessarily die but to either get the attention of people to understand their pain or to "escape" the extreme emotions they feel. Another point is acting on impulse, many times people with a borderline personality disorder "don't know" how they even got to attempting suicide. For most, it's a rush of poor impulsivity, anxiety, and urgency to "stop this now!" Suicidal gestures can be used to show that they are suffering or to get their way. I've had patients with borderline personality disorder who were on psychiatric holds yell and scream at me that if I didn't let them out right away, they would kill themselves, and it would be my fault for them doing it. You can see the external locus of control here, "I'm *not* in control of my actions, if *you* hold me in here, I will *kill* myself because *you* won't let me go." Notice there is no concept of control for the actual behavior of trying to kill one's self; it is merely a repercussion of my action to not letting her go.

Sometimes you may get a call with the person with borderline personality disorder stating they just overdosed on pills. You get them to the emergency room only to find out that they ingested about three pills of Tylenol, by far not even close to fatal dosages. Should their suicidal statements be taken seriously? As frequent and frustrating as they can be, the answer is yes. Why? Because people with borderline can complete suicide, and it's mostly done by pushing that line a little too far. You see, surviving a suicide attempt can be thrilling for some. You just survived an event meant to kill you. This renews hope, renews importance, turns the "reset" button on for some. But even most distorted is the feeling of control that comes from this. "I survived this uncontrollable event, which means I actually have control over it." Unfortunately, this to someone with borderline personality is like heroin, highly addictive.

The last piece of the borderline triad is an obvious part due to what you have just read above: turbulent interpersonal relationships. People with borderline personality disorders tend to have conflict in almost every personal relationship they have. It doesn't matter who it is, parent, significant other, coworker, you name it! At times it's not obvious, maybe the focus is elsewhere for the time being, but if the person feels any importance in the relationship, it takes new meaning to those with a borderline personality disorder. In some regards, trauma begets trauma. Time and time again, we see people who were abused as children grow up only to be abused again and again. In borderline personality disorder, there is a seeking of strong, controlling, and confident people. This is exactly the kind of person they want to emulate and be a part of to feel safe and secure. It just so happens to be that many abusive significant others display all these qualities. Mix this in with an emotionally unstable and emotionally demanding person, and you have the perfect recipe for more trauma. They seek these qualities because of their intense fear of abandonment. Being alone is torture to someone with borderline because their meaning is found in others. People with borderline personality disorder tend to push the limits and manipulate people in their personal circle. It seems odd for someone who has an extreme fear of abandonment to push and push their loved one so far that that loved one may just cut off all ties, but there's a double edge sword here. It is easy for anyone to say, "I love you" and "I'll support you" when everything is fine, dandy, and stable. The real test of "I love you" and "I'll support you" is if you will indeed be there for me even though I've been terrible to you. That really shows support and dedication. Unfortunately, most people won't put up with that, only to lead the person with a borderline personality disorder to have their self-fulfilled prophecy, that the person was not there for them, they were abandoned, they are not "lovable," they are useless, etc. This sends people with borderline into a perpetual circle of reinforcement that is very hard to break because it all seems so true to them overtime.

Fortunately, treatment is available for borderline personality disorder. Although most people with a borderline personality disorder don't see what they do as being disordered. Marsha Linehan created a widely used, highly evidential, psychotherapy called *Dialectical Behavioural Therapy* or DBT. This therapy is a combination of cognitive behavioral therapy (CBT), mindfulness practice, and emotional tolerance building. DBT has been shown to decrease self-harm and suicidal behaviors in those who take it. DBT typically consists of individual sessions and group sessions to help tailor specific issues but also to see other people's patterns of thought to gain insight into the disorder. DBT is also useful for other mental health disorders, such as depression, trauma, anxiety, and more. Medications have at best modest effect for people with a borderline personality disorder. Medications are typically aimed for depression and suicidal thoughts and also targeted for impulse control. In general, borderline personality disorder tends to be one of the most frequently seen personality disorders (around 6% of the general population) and is one of the most "visible" to those who know people with a borderline personality disorder. Understanding how the borderline mind operates is key to understanding how to communicate and ultimately help those with a borderline personality disorder.

Histrionic

Histrionic stems from the word, *histrio*, which stems from the Latin word for "actor." Indeed, people with histrionic personality disorder have a pervasive pattern of attention-seeking, negative or positive. If someone with a histrionic personality disorder is not the center of attention in a social setting, extreme measures will be taken to get the attention onto them. This can include exaggeration of feelings and emotions, the push for "my story is more important and more entertaining than yours," and if these tactics don't work, then they can display intense emotions with crying, tantrums, and accusations of other people even though the facts may be abhorrently wrong. Stories or explanations maybe not only exaggerated but lacking in detail to avoid the finding out of the truth of the situation. If questioned, an array of even more lacking details may follow, thus, exhausting the questioner. People with a histrionic personality disorder may use sexual seduction to gain their attention. This can be through elusive flirtation to seductive clothing styles. This ongoing narrative of attention-seeking is constant as it gives them that superficial reassurance that will surely run out as soon as the attention is gone.

Because of the superficial nature of attention-seeking, relationships with people with histrionic personality disorder tend to be minimal, shallow, or in complete disarray, although they will tend to over-exaggerate the intimacy of these relationships. They want to be known as "the go-getters," "the life of the party," and crave for people to admire them and their "lifestyle." Indeed, social media becomes an obsession for some as it is a platform to filter all the events and qualities about yourself to others without much threat to have to defend yourself in light of these postings. Depression and anxiety can be common in people with a histrionic personality disorder. The strong need to be dependent on constant attention, the emptiness that follows, and absolute despair if they don't get the attention can bleed into depressive episodes. Because of the nature of all personality disorders, this source of depression and anxiety will be very hard for the person to tell that their behaviors are a determinant to these consequences, so there is a tendency to blame others for these feelings of inadequacy, low self-esteem, and boredom.

Like other personality disorders, people with histrionic personality rarely, if ever, seek treatment. Their behaviors and actions are completely in line with their view of how the world works and see other people as trying to play the game as well. Indeed, people with a histrionic personality disorder may call other people "histrionic" because they feel threatened and over exaggerate people's behaviors. For the few that end up in therapy, it mostly becomes a new stage for their performance, leaving the therapist to tend to emotional exaggerations, off-topic grandeur events, and the apparent lack of detail that is hard to ground. Expectedly, most people with a histrionic personality disorder will never touch the mental health system and will remain very high functioning.

Narcissistic

Narcissism is probably one of the most known words in all of mental health. Indeed, it is thrown around to many types of people in certain areas, mostly politics, academics, and doctors. Narcissism comes from the Greek mythology of Narcissus, the hunter from Thespiae. The Greek story tells of Narcissus discovering his reflection in a still pool. Enamored and infatuated with his beauty, he could not break his stare. The fire of passion felt inside from his own beauty, and self-love consumed him, burning Narcissus into a gold and white flower, which we call the daffodil (genus name: *narcissus*) flower we see today. Like the story, people with narcissistic personality disorder have a constant obsession with their self-perceived great qualities. Their grandiose thinking makes them feel superior to others in regard to talent, beauty, and ability to get away with anything. Not only do they feel superior, but they may also believe that they are a part of a small elite or superior group, usually consisting of other narcissists or subordinates enamored by the narcissistic person. Of course, offspring from the person with narcissistic personality disorder are included in this special group, which will entail the children learning that they are exceptional and superior to others.

Interestingly, unlike antisocial personality disorder, narcissists have incredibly fragile self-esteem. They are incredibly sensitive to any criticism and tend to react by lashing out and trying to "destroy" the source of criticism. Enragement is a common tool used to squash criticism. Lack of empathy is very strong. Those they hurt are just "jealous" of their narcissistic abilities. Like antisocial personality disorder, they see every interaction as an "I win, you lose" type mentality with the belief that everyone else knows and plays the same game. Having narcissism can wreak havoc on interpersonal relationships and future prospects, but it can also be a massive aid to achieving fame and high positions of power due to the exuberant confidence they can display. Indeed, many people in politics, medicine, law, celebrities, CEOs, and other positions of high power have narcissistic tendencies that aided their progression to these positions and titles. It is evident that many of us will come across people with narcissism as they tend to be around 1-6% of the general population, depending on the statistics you look at.

Narcissistic personality disorder may be one of the hardest personality disorders to get any treatment for. Once again, they are great, and you are not, so why are you telling them they need help? For someone with a narcissistic personality disorder, going into therapy is just asking for them to dig past their present superficiality into areas where they are vulnerable. It is hard for anyone to be vulnerable; it is damn near impossible for a person with a narcissistic personality disorder to be vulnerable. The few times in my professional life I have seen bona fide people with narcissism in therapy was due to threats of divorce or the leaving of a relationship. And even then, their intention was not going there because they wanted to be in the loving relationship and they care about their significant other. It was mostly because a divorce or separation would hurt their ego or may hurt their image in whatever field they work in. To get any "buy-in" they will have to feel as though they will "win' in the end.

Anxious

Obsessive Compulsive

But wait, there's an obsessive-compulsive *disorder* AND obsessive-compulsive *personality disorder*? Yes, and it can be confusing I admit. Once again, it stems from how personality disorders present: stable, persistent, and generally not as imparting as mood or thought disorders. Somebody with obsessive-compulsive personality disorder has a very rigid need for order or cleanliness. They may be the types that will wear surgical shoe covers while in the house or spend an extra 2 hours on a paper to make sure it contains precision that they demand. They tend to love rules, lists for everything, devotion to a craft or work, and even value systems. The obsessive and compulsive nature of their personality is seen as a huge pro rather than a con, and they may say that this way of being is what has led to any successes they have experienced. People with obsessive-compulsive *disorder* on the other hand, typically have impairments and inability to move forward on life goals due to the strong intrusive thoughts and behaviors. People with the disorder tend to know or will eventually admit that this is a hindrance and a problem in their life. Treatment, like many of the other personality disorders, is generally not sought. If treatment were to be an option, it tends to be more towards the therapy side, including cognitive behavioral therapy and other types of behavioral therapies. Anti-depressants (SSRIs specifically) have shown minor to modest improvement.

Dependent

A dependent personality disorder is, once again, a rarer personality disorder (roughly 0.5% of the population). Generally, people with dependent personality disorder rely heavily on others (most of the time a significant other) for emotional and psychological needs. This can also be for physical needs, as well. This is different than say a person who is physically handicapped and relies on their significant other or family for support. People with dependent personality disorder tend to have great functionality and ability to achieve high functioning; it's just they tend to be scared and frightened of such independence. Having a secure and stabilized person to rely on is incredibly comforting, even at the expense of extreme submission or possible abuse from whoever they rely on. They tend to be extremely passive, have *analysis paralysis* where they analyze any problem to the point of being paralyzed and never doing anything about the problem. They tend to come from backgrounds of the extremes, neglect or over-authoritarian parenting, or long abusive relationships. Generally, therapy is the key to helping people with a dependent personality disorder with the goal of finding independence and coping with anxiety when decisions need to be made. Medications can help the anxiety symptoms but generally don't help the situation or the behaviors seen in dependent personality disorder. Therapy is key to this personality disorder.

Avoidant

Avoidant personality disorder tends to be a more frequent personality disorder, affecting about 2-3% of the general population, depending on the statistics you use. It strikes both males and females equally. The "avoidance" part of avoidant personality disorder is avoiding social situations and interactions. There is an excessive feeling of being inept at communicating and engaging with others. The feeling is so strong that they tend to avoid any social situation. Fear of being humiliated, "found out," rejected, or not liked, they tend to choose jobs that don't involve interactions with others and are generally independent. When you talk to people with avoidant personality disorder about what it would look like to NOT be socially inept, they will tend to give you a glamorized, over the top, and unachievable view. This leads to a thought that they will never measure up and be at that level, despite the reality that nobody will be at that level. They tend to have intense shyness and fear of abandonment. Substance use can be used to self-cope with the anxiety and fear involved in social interactions. Causes are very complicated and not well understood. There tends to be a push towards childhood temperament of shyness and quietness, coupled with likely events of being made fun of or humiliated in childhood that solidifies their view and persona to the outside world.

Treatment can be beneficial, which is not as common for other personality disorders. Increasing social skills and using cognitive behavioral therapy are key treatments. The biggest barriers are trust and openness. Unlike other personality disorders, people with avoidant personality disorder tend to have some inclination that things may not be at their best and know that they are not well. This can lead the way to open those conversations of trying different treatments.

6

EATING DISORDERS

"I may not be in control of anything else, but I am in control of my body."
-Karen Carpenter

Anorexia Nervosa

Prevalence: around 1% - 4% of the general population in women, 0.3% in men

Signs and Symptoms

- Restriction of food intake with subsequent weight loss or failure to maintain a healthy weight
- Intense fear of being "fat" or having weight gain
- Distorted thoughts about themselves and of eating
- Seeing their underweight body and perceiving themselves as "fat."
- Believing there is no problem
- Believes eating a meal will lead to significant weight gain
- Amenorrhea - dysregulated or complete stopping of the menstrual cycle
- Lanugo - soft, fine hair on face or body

- Excessive exercise
- Food rituals – such as cutting food into little pieces
- Intolerance to cold
- Fatigue
- Brittle hair, brittle nails, yellowish skin

Brain Function

Anorexia nervosa has been classically seen as a psychologically-based illness with heavy physical consequences. To understand anorexia is to understand its close relationship with obsessive-compulsive disorder (OCD). Indeed, the brain chemical, serotonin, is implicated in both anorexia and OCD. Although serotonin is implicated, this may be more related as a contributing factor of the anxiety, obsessiveness, and appetite decrease side of anorexia instead of being the brain chemical responsible for anorexia. Most of the anorexia behaviors are learned and practiced, not necessarily "inflicted" by serotonin deregulation. Some neuroimaging studies have shown that the area of the brain that helps us with introspection (the ability to see our own mental and emotional processes) is altered, which also determines our control of cognitive, or thinking abilities.

Through Their Eyes

Anorexia nervosa is likened to obsessive thoughts and compulsive actions; thus, people who have anorexia feel a constant battle in their heads regarding the way they perceive their body. The strong intrusive thoughts of "you are fat," "you are ugly," "you are gross," are constant and reinforced. Like OCD, people with anorexia tend to have perfectionist tendencies. Trying to create order and control is relieving to the uncontrolled thoughts and behaviors that inflict someone with anorexia. Frustration and anger are not even adequate words to describe the relentless view of yourself going through the starvation and purging behaviors, while saying, "Stop! Don't do this!" This typically leads to an increased shame spiral, which reinforces the idea that no one will "get you" because even you don't "get you." This can lead to the tendency to hide these behaviors as the strong sense of shame leads to a fear of being "found out" or "judged" and, most importantly, not understood. The idea of treatment is frightening because the very thing you feel you want control over will be taken away from you (anorexia treatment involves strict regiments around eating, including weighing and monitoring). This makes treatment seem like a nightmare of embarrassment and more shame, which leads to a "damned if you do, damned if you don't" because shame and embarrassment are already so encompassing. Most survivors and those who come out of anorexia nervosa, if trusting, will tell you that, while the behaviors of starvation or purging may be gone, intrusive thoughts of "being fat" and "not being thin enough" linger for years. While these may be distressing and intrusive, treatment aims to disarm the incredible power they have, which ultimately will help reduce the urge, or compulsive, to starve or purge.

Treatment: Psychotherapy, Anti-Depressants, Mood Stabilizers

Bulimia Nervosa

Prevalence: 0.5% of the general population (U.S.) 5 times higher in females than in males

Signs and Symptoms

- Repeating binge eating episodes, typically each episode being 2 hours or less
- Following binge episodes, intense and intrusive thoughts to do a drastic measure to not gain weight from the binge episode

- Drastic measure is purging (vomiting)
- Fixations on weight, calories, exercise

Physical signs including:

- Dehydration
- Gastric reflux
- Electrolyte disruptions
- Inflamed throat (esophagitis)
- Calluses on knuckles (from vomiting)
- Dental erosion
- High heart rate
- Low blood pressure
- Digestion issues (constipation, diarrhea, peptic ulcers)

Brain Function

In many ways, bulimia nervosa is similar to anorexia nervosa in regard to biological and genetic factors. Serotonin (feel-good brain chemical) is implicated for bulimia nervosa. There is extensive evidence of bulimia having a genetic component, and it runs in families. Similarly, growing up in a household where role models fixate on weight and calories teach the genetically vulnerable person to hyper-focus on image and appearance, often leading to the body image distortions seen. Bulimia and anorexia both reinforce the behaviors by not eating enough or receiving enough of a chemical tryptophan, which is found in meats and other foods. Tryptophan is an ingredient for serotonin, which is already lowered with bulimia and anorexia, thus not eating or purging keeps the person in a state that intensifies anorexia or bulimia. There is a focus on bulimia and poly cystic ovarian syndrome (PCOS) as PCOS disrupts estrogen and testosterone regulation. Both estrogen and testosterone are important in weight maintaining. Interestingly, people with

PCOS tend to be more overweight or average weight compared to anorexia, and a usual sign of PCOS is also being overweight and having difficulty losing weight.

Through Their Eyes

Bulimia nervosa is a very challenging eating disorder (all eating disorders are!) to treat. Many times, a person with bulimia has pretty good insight and knows that these behaviors are impairing and taxing on their health. Yet the strong and intrusive thoughts of maintaining ideal weights (typically unrealistic) and trying to maintain rigid, restrictive type diets seem out of control and defeating. As with many eating disorders, a strong sense to harness control and create predictability is at the heart of bulimia. A general thought pattern is, "If I can't even control myself, then I'm very out of control," which is terrifying. Indeed, trying to control the very things you eat and expecting certain results from these actions creates the illusion that you are in control when in reality, you are being controlled by the unrealistic expectations and goals.

Distorted thoughts about their self-image lead to distorted ideas about what to do, which then leads to distorted behaviors to try and remedy the distorted thoughts. This is what perpetuates the binge-purge cycle; the unrealistic goals reach the breaking point, and the person feels that they cannot hold the pattern anymore. With a binge episode, it is likened to dissociation or being out of contact with reality. The mind almost doesn't have any time to think about what is going on before it's too late and 5000 - 15000 calories have been consumed. By the time the person realizes the binging, extreme guilt and shame are very overbearing. Guilt, shame, and secrecy are seen as prime ingredients for someone with bulimia. These also feed into each other into an endless loop, making the sufferer feel as if there will never be an option for anything different. For a person with bulimia, being offered treatment or support seems genuine but not feasible because of the engrained thoughts of being "defective." These can be even more complicated as many people with eating disorders suffer from trauma. Remember, a traumatic experience makes the person feel out of control. The body's response is to do any soothing behaviors to give the feeling that you are, indeed, in control, even if detrimental to your overall health.

Treatment: Psychotherapy, Anti-Depressants, Mood Stabilizers, Anti-Anxiety

Binge Eating Disorder

Prevalence: 1-3% of the general population

Signs and Symptoms

- Eating a large amount of food not typically eaten by most people and typically within a 2 hour or less period
- Feelings of being out of control
- Uncomfortable eating around others
- Secretive or off-hour binges (2 am etc.)
- Isolation, eating alone, avoiding discussions regarding food
- Frequent diet changes or diet fads
- Profound feelings of depression, low self-esteem, disgust, and guilt
- Weight fluctuating and tendency to be overweight

Brain Function

Like other eating disorders, binge eating tends to be more of a "symptom" of underlying emotional problems. Typically, depression and its ugly head of shame, low self-esteem, body dissatisfaction, and internalized worthlessness is a common underlying issue. Depression, thus, is the fuel to the fire of binge eating. Evidence points to a high genetic probability for binge eating, with some estimates up to 50% probability. Yet, like other eating disorders, there are environmental components, such as child abuse or negative childhood experiences. This makes sense when looking at the brain and how it responds to stressors and depression. In many ways, binge eating is a coping mechanism that raises the brain chemical dopamine, which makes you feel good and motivates you to do it again. From an evolutionary standpoint, eating foods (especially fats) increases serotonin (which is low in depression). Guess what? Low serotonin also makes you impulsive and anxious, which can explain why binge eating episodes appear to be out of control. All these factors accumulate and reinforce each other to make binge eating incredibly hard to control.

Tips and Wisdom

Binge eating disorder, like other eating disorders, stems from poor self-image. With constant feedback from the media, peers, and role models, the constant pressure to look certain ways is very apparent and real. Binge eating disorder is the most common eating disorder in the United States. The binges are generally seen as a coping mechanism gone wild. As stated above, depression is a common underlying disturbance in binge eating disorder, and when depression and feelings of despair hit new lows, eating (especially fats and sugars) can give immediate relief to those feelings. In many ways, the underlying emotional issues (depression, anxiety) are the factors that lead to the coping (although maladaptive) mechanism of binge eating or any other eating disorder. If you suspect a loved one has binge eating disorder or disturbances, monitor the food amounts in your home, observe for fluctuating diets, and fluctuating weights. Increased difficulties in work due to poor concentration from binge eating all night or preoccupied with shame and guilt from binging may be apparent. As always, I approached loved ones with binge eating with delicacy. Many times, this may be the biggest darkest secret they have. Simply saying that it is happening is incredibly brave. Validate their reasoning and viewpoints of binge eating, allow the natural discovery of underlying depression and anxiety, and then acknowledge those components. A lot of times, people with eating disorders fixate on the eating disorder when shifting the concern to underlying depression, and anxiety can provide new insight and potential hope

Treatment: Psychotherapy, Anti-Depressants. FDA approved Vyvanse (lisdexamfetamine)

7

PTSD AND OTHER MENTAL DISORDERS

"Courage is resistance to fear, mastery of fear, not absence of fear."
–Mark Twain

Post-Traumatic Stress Disorder (PTSD)

Prevalence: around 3% of the general population

Signs and Symptoms

- Experiencing or witnessing death, threatened death or serious injury, including physical, emotional, or sexual violence
- Very intrusive thoughts or memories about the traumatic event
- Recurring nightmares related to the traumatic event
- Dissociation or flashbacks
- Distress when reminded of the event
- Physical "revving" up (tension, high heart rate, rapid breathing)
- Avoidance or efforts to avoid any triggers or situations that may cause distress
- Triggers - an unexpected reminder of the traumatic event causing

instant distress (includes people, places, activities, discussions, objects, or situations)
- Difficulty recalling details of the traumatic event
- Shame, guilt, feelings of being "defective" or "bad," self-blame
- Negative views of the world or environment
- Lessened pleasure in activities that were once pleasurable
- Isolation and detachment from others (including loved ones and family)
- Difficulty expressing positive emotions (smiling, laughing)
- Irritability and aggressiveness
- Reckless and impulsive behaviors
- Hyper-vigilant or hyper-focus on the environment for "dangers."
- Overactive startle response - startles easily
- Difficulty concentrating
- Insomnia or sleep disturbances

Brain Function

A traumatic event or series of traumatic events wreak havoc on the brain. The brain's primary purpose, first and foremost, is survival. The brain is primed to keep you alive. To do this, it has a very sensitive fear detection system, which is called the *limbic system*. Traumatic experiences activate this part of the brain and strengthen it like a muscle. With a traumatic event, your brain learns to keep a heightened lookout to prevent any trauma from happening again. The only unfortunate part is that with such a strong limbic system, your body and emotions are incredibly uncomfortable. Like a muscle, the limbic system is strong and overactive, and you are constantly stuck in the famous fight or flight, which is geared for our survival. With the brain's fear center on active duty, the part of the brain that helps us make decisions, socialize, and control our impulses (prefrontal cortex) goes to the back burner. To the traumatic brain, another trauma can happen at any time, and anywhere, so socializing or spending time thinking about actions is not an option. This hypersensitivity in the brain leads to the hyper-focus on the environment, the highly distressing triggers that can send a person with PTSD into a frenzy. The brain doesn't care about false alarms, but the person has to go through the suffering of the constant amped up alarm system. With the brain being so easily triggered and hypersensitive, people with PTSD try to avoid any such triggers or distressing thoughts as they don't want to go through the woes of another traumatic experience.

Through Their Eyes

PTSD presents in many ways in different types of populations. If you could put three words that are universal in PTSD, they would be shame, exhausting, and terrifying. Shame is what keeps the secrecy in PTSD, and those with PTSD feel that talking to others about their trauma will be futile. There are tremendous feelings of isolation in PTSD. There is a sense that no one understands them and that people are not trustworthy. Add onto that the horrible feelings that come with discussing the traumatic event, and you have a perfect concoction of repression of traumatic memories and isolative tendencies. Because most traumas involve being traumatized by another human (unless it's a weather catastrophe or similar), trust is obliterated. Everything is in question now because humans are capable of some pretty terrible things. Strangers, especially, are a big threat. Being at a party or a social gathering with strangers is not only terrifying but very exhausting. PTSD is also exhausting because of its relentlessness. Many with PTSD feel that they can never "rest" from the PTSD symptoms. Even in your sleep, the one thing that is supposed to restore you, is your enemy. Poor sleep and the terrifying nightmares keep the trauma alive. People with PTSD get so exhausted that ideas of death or suicide are common. The hopelessness and social isolation carry huge effects of depression. Feelings of inadequacy and "defectiveness" are a common theme, making progressions in jobs, schooling, or other obligations very hard and challenging.

Treatment: Psychotherapy, Anti-Depressants, Mood Stabilizers, Anti-

Anxiety, Antipsychotics

Other Noteworthy Mental Illnesses: Explained Briefly

While there is a multitude of different mental illnesses, each having its own significance and importance, we cannot go through every one of them. My goal in this book has been to outline and discuss the most frequent and most impairing of the illnesses. This section discusses other mental illnesses that are seen, but for the purposes of this book, it will be presented in a synopsis style.

Dissociative Identity Disorder (formerly Multiple Personality Disorder)

A relatively "popular" mental illness in the media, dissociative identity disorder (DID) consists of the presence of two or more alter personalities or personality states. Of course, what you see in the movies is not a very good presentation of DID. DID almost always results from extreme trauma, mostly in the childhood years. People with DID typically not only have experienced trauma but have experienced it in many ways and typically ongoing. Physical, sexual, emotional, and neglect are a typical combination. What you see when this happens is the person is not able to establish a sense of "self." So, in many ways, they don't understand who "they" are in a sense. While the personality alters can range greatly, there tends to be a personality that is almost angelic, perfect, innocent, and naive. This serves to help comfort those feelings of being "dirty" or "sexualized" by the abuse. On the same token, you may see a personality alter that is "evil," meaning dirty, highly sexualized, violent, manipulative, aggressive and more. This may allow the person to express the feelings in a way that has no constraint.

To further clarify, let's look at a famous movie, *Forrest Gump*. In this movie, Jenny runs with Forrest into the cornfields when Jenny's drunk father starts slamming doors and yelling at Jenny to come over to him. What the audience learns is that Jenny is a victim of her father's drunken abuse, mostly sexual. When she and Forrest get far enough away, she immediately gets on the ground and starts praying to be a bird so she can fly "far far away." At that moment, the imagination of being a bird that can get away at a moment's notice is very comforting and provides some buffer to the horrendous reality she faces daily. In DID, that same mechanism of imagination is haywire and creates a personality where the person alternates into that role. It's not escapism as the person has no control over this. It is the brain's way of trying to provide natural relief from the distressing memories and fear that exist.

Treatment for DID involves very heavy psychotherapy for the trauma, although most people with DID will always have elements of the disorder. DID is common with PTSD, but also an array of personality disorders as a lot of personality disorders have a high background in traumatic events. It's also important to know that DID is very rare. Some claim to have DID but really may have a personality disorder that presents with a poor self-concept (borderline personality disorder). This is not to say that they don't suffer, but merely that the disorders, once again, are not cookie cutter, and they merge and overlap in many ways.

Factitious Disorder (Munchausen's)

Although rare, factitious disorder, formerly known as Munchausen's, makes headline news and grabs the attention of many when hearing about this disorder. Factitious disorder is simulating, inducing, or aggravating a medical condition to get attention and empathy. Such acts may be injecting one's self with insulin to dramatically lower blood sugar and then going to the hospital to claim that they have diabetes. Digestive symptoms and odd, unexplainable pains may be very common, as well. It tends to run very high in white, middle-aged males. The cause is very poorly understood.

Probably more infamous and frenzied by the media is factitious disorder by proxy or *Munchausen's by proxy*. This involves, typically mothers, who intentionally induce symptoms of illness onto another person, most of the time, their child. Many reasons for this are understood. One is relief from caretaker responsibilities, or it may be getting sympathy indirectly from the child's suffering. In some cases, it is to "be a hero" and "catch" a dying person just in the nick of time. This is sometimes seen by nurses who purposely give or merely watch their patients decompensate and then intervene at the last moment to become "the hero".

As such, this disorder is not very well understood, and there is no consensus as to the underlying factors that increase the risk of Munchausen's. Treatment is rather limited as well and typically focuses on psychotherapy of underlying issues of self-inadequacy.

Intermittent Explosive Disorder (IED)

Intermittent explosive disorder, IED, involves episodes of extreme, out of proportion, aggressive impulsions. Although you may see highly impulsive and agitated episodes in some mental disorders, IED occurs when there is no other mental disorder present or causing the episodes. Many with IED explain the episodes in almost a "trance" like state or utter out of control anger. When experiencing IED, between episodes of intense anger, there is a general calm and good impulse control. Indeed, many with IED feel tremendous guilt and remorse when the episode is done as they feel tremendous amounts of shame from being so out of control. As a matter of fact, early research into IED sought to search for organic brain disease as these agitated episodes were almost mimicking a seizure in that it was completely out of control and random. IED is more common in men and tends to have a higher propensity to strike physically large men who feel incompetent, dependent, or not masculine. Traumatic backgrounds are very common as there is an intense fear of being humiliated. Typically, treatment consists of psychopharmacological medications that help with impulse control and psychotherapy designed to help bring awareness to triggers and underlying feelings about themselves.

Complicated Bereavement and Grief

Losing a loved one is incredibly difficult. In many ways, it's not only missing their companionship but also triggers that deep fear of what it means to die and what happens to "you." Grieving is as complex as the uniqueness and individuality of us all. So how can we determine what is "complicated" or "prolonged" grieving when it is so unique to the individual? I, too, struggle with this concept and diagnosis as I feel that I can never understand the circumstances behind the grieving of a loved one enough to make a clinical diagnosis that they "should be able to be more functioning by x date." Nonetheless, a different perspective is that we distinguish complicated grief based on impairment, not to tell people that they need to be functioning or uplifted by "x" date, but to develop ways of helping those who are struggling and having massive impairments in their everyday life.

Grieving those who have passed typically follows a fashion of denial, anger, bargaining, depression, and acceptance, as specified by Kübler-Ross. Indeed, these stages don't go in order, nor do they go from one to the next. You may be depressed one day, denial stage next week, and back to depression again. Typically, what specifies "complicated" grief is an extreme impairment in any one of these stages. This could be a parent who lost a child two years ago who is in complete denial and not accepting that their child has passed. It can be constant talk or yearning to be with the loved one years later with an inability to focus on daily tasks and enjoying their years alive. Survivor's guilt is very common, where the person feels that it should have been them who passed away, not their loved one. Strong desires to die and be with their loved one or isolating from others to protect themselves from another loved one dying is also very common. Confusion and feeling meaningless encapsulate why their bodies cannot move forward.

Treatment for complicated grief includes psychotherapy and grief counseling. Be aware that most of the time, if a person with complicated grief is seeking treatment, it's typically for sleep issues related to the grief. It is also important to know that giving medications that alleviate anxiety or depression may interfere with the mourning process as it doesn't allow the body to go through the motions of acceptance.

Medical Conditions That Can Mimic Mental Disorders

Medical Conditions With Psychiatric Symptoms			
Anxiety	Depression and Suicidal Thoughts	Hallucinations & Delusions	Confusion or Memory Issues
Hyperthyroidism	Hypothyroidism	Insomnia	Dementia
Lyme Disease	Hyperparathyroidism	Parkinsons	Alzheimers
Brain Tumours	Cushing's Syndrome	Brain Tumour	Encephalopathy
Dementias	Addison's Disease	HIV	Strokes
Alzheimers	Multiple Sclerosis	Seizures/Epilepsy	Meningitis
	Hepatitis	Strokes	Encephalitis
	Traumatic Brain Injury		Traumatic Brain Injury
	Electrolyte Disturbances		Brain Tumour
	Lewy Body Dementia		Hypothyroidism
	Encephalopathy		

Table 2.3 Medical Conditions with Psychiatric Components

It is always important to remember that our brain is not a separate entity from our bodies. We are finely intricate and interwoven machines. Indeed, some medical conditions can present as a mental disorder, and ruling out these medical conditions is an important part of the journey to find the best treatment and best outcomes for you and your loved one.

8

THE MEDICATIONS

"The harder the conflict, the greater the triumph"
-**George Washington**

Goals of Treatment

Treatment takes on many faces and is very personal to each person. While some providers may argue that their methodology is superior, in reality, each modality has its strengths and weaknesses. Also, each mental condition responds better or more thoroughly with different modalities. For some, medications may be the optimum route, others it may be therapy and complementary alternative therapy. As a nurse practitioner who prescribes, my brain tends to lean towards medications because that's what most of my training and practice consists of. It isn't that I'm biased against other modalities of treatment, merely that my knowledge base is stronger in that area. If you were to read a book similar to this book from an author who is a therapist, you wouldn't expect a massive portion of the book being about medications, but rather more therapy based.

Nonetheless, my aim is to not only give information about medications, but also therapy and complementary alternative therapies. All are equal and have effectiveness. Treatment is always personal and tailored to the needs of the person. The goal of treatment should always aim for the remission of symptoms. Striving for the best outcome is a good goal to have. If residual symptoms still linger, treatment should be geared to trying to maintain those symptoms. With the goal of remission, we must also recognize that certain mental conditions are very treatment-resistant and may not make it to full remission. This is mostly due to medications not being the best yet and needing more research. It may also be many factors related to different therapies not being as effective as others. It could be the person with a mental condition creating some barriers to treatment. Whatever the case is, this is a reality of treatment, and it's a journey that is challenging, yet profound.

When engaging treatment, always try to remember not to fall into the "doing okay syndrome," where you or your loved one state they are "doing okay" in order to not let down the provider who is putting work into bettering their lives. I see this often where my patients are sincere and polite in telling me that my medication regimen or therapy interventions are doing well, when, in reality, they are minimally working, or honestly, downright not working at all. Honesty about your symptoms is crucial to refining treatment and further aiming for that goal of remission. Will we, as a team, be able to solve every issue? No, but then again, that's not generally what people are looking for. Getting to be functional and having a purpose in life is usually the main goal of people.

Do I need medications or therapy?

For the best results? Typically, both! But in reality, it depends on the person and the mental condition. Indeed, some mental illnesses are biologically based, while others may be more psychologically based. Of course, both biology and psychology intermingle, but depending on the person's circumstances and driving factor in their mental illness, it can fall from one side to the other. For some general information, typically, any mental illness with psychosis - hallucinations, delusions - will need medications. This is due to psychosis being a strong biological brain-based issue. Do people with psychosis not take medications? Of course, but they have a much tougher road ahead and generally will relapse more and more. For anxiety and depression, once again, it depends. If a person is anxious and depressed because they witnessed their husband get killed, then therapy may be the best option initially. If a person is depressed and lying in bed all day for no particular reason or stressor, that may be more biologically based depression. This can get complicated of course. Take panic disorder. Panic disorder has a lot of research about its biological disruptions, including a hypersensitive alarm system that is hard to turn off. Medications are very useful in panic disorder. But! Panic disorder responds very well to cognitive behavioral therapy (CBT). It responds so well that most people who do CBT for panic disorder will never have a panic attack again. So once again, it depends on the person and the mental illness. Bipolar disorder almost always needs medications. The throws of mania and depression are exhausting and debilitating. Add that around 15% of people with bipolar disorder will die from suicide and this places a priority on medications that help keep the mood stable. Whatever the case is, always feel free to try one modality first, then maybe another one if results are not optimal. Research demonstrates that medications AND therapy not only fair better than one alone, but they are actually synergistic, meaning that they enhance each other much more than if the modality is done alone. Always be open to the options and find that personalized treatment that is as unique as you or your loved one is.

Do I need medications forever?

This is a very common question I get and rightfully so. Nobody plans on taking medication for their whole life. Then again, nobody plans on taking medications period. The answer to this question is (drumroll) it depends.

Ambiguity strikes again. But there are some factors that determine if a medication is taken for situational distress or the long haul. Schizophrenia or any mental illness that has psychosis will almost always need medications for a lifetime. These are very brain-based illnesses that have chemical disturbances. Are there people with psychotic disorders that don't take medications and are able to function? Yes, but we are talking about a sliver of the vast majority who need to take medications to remain functional. Bipolar disorder is another illness that regularly needs lifelong medication management depending on the severity. Bipolar is a lifelong illness, unlike depression or anxiety, which can be lifelong or clearly situational. For depression, anxiety, and trauma disorders, medications may or may not be a part of treatment. They may be used for situational depression (say the death of a child) or not used at all for the same circumstance. Panic disorder and many anxiety disorders tend to start with medications, but when therapy is covered and practiced, the medications will be discontinued.

If you or a loved one is taking medications and there is a decision to stop medications, always ask yourself, "Do I feel better because my situation in life is better, or is it because the medication is working and keeping my mood in check?" A lot of times, I have somebody tell me that they want to stop their antidepressants because they "feel better". It is most likely because the antidepressant is working. Take it away, and you may not feel better. In general, the number of mood episodes can determine if a medication will be lifelong or not. For example, someone goes through a major depressive episode, and it's their first one. They start an antidepressant and stay on it for the recommended 9-12 months and then discontinue it. If another major depressive episode occurs, you'll restart the medication and, this time, continue it for the recommended 1-2 years then discontinue it. If you have a third major depressive episode, then that's a sign that this will be a probable lifelong medication regimen. Another good rule of thumb is the longer the disorder has been occurring; the longer the treatment should be. In general, untreated mental illnesses tend to become more treatment-resistant over time and cause more permanency. Someone who has had major depression for 18 years will need longer treatment than a person who has major depression for three months.

Medications: Worse than the U.S. political divide

They always say don't talk about religion, sex, or politics with strangers. Might as well add views of psychiatric medications with that. Psychiatric medications carry a lot of meaning behind them. It's one thing to take blood pressure medication. What does that say about you to others? Your blood pressure is high? You may eat too much salt? Nothing too harsh. Now tell someone you take Haldol or Prozac. What's the response? You're crazy? Out of control? Weak? Nuts? Dumb? Dangerous? These hit straight at who you are as a person and your character. You are being stigmatized. These medications are like a loaded gun, ready and cocked to cause trouble. Such powerful meanings and stigma turn people off from psychiatric medications. Images in our thoughts of being "zombies" or "flat" come to mind. Sedated not to feel anymore. My grandmother believed that psychiatrists promoted divorces and gave medications to numb the feeling of love.

In honesty, psychiatric medications are no different than any other medication. All medications have side effects, just like street drugs, alcohol, and, yes, natural products. Yes, we should reserve medications for mental illness that hasn't responded to therapy or other treatments, but unfortunately, that is not reality. The same is for every person with high blood pressure.

Could you imagine giving a blood pressure medication after having them try intensive exercise and dieting with sodium monitoring only to see if that fails first? That's okay if the patient agrees to do that, but we know that a lot of people won't or physically cannot do that. Holding the blood pressure medication saves them from potential side effects but robs them of protecting their organs and heart from the damage of high blood pressure.

The same can be said of psychosis and mania episodes. Psychotic episodes get worse over time if not treated. The brain trying to keep regulation will keep breaking down with each psychotic episode, thus raising the patient's baseline higher and higher. This is why sometimes we see people with mental illness on the streets in a constant psychotic state. They may have tons of medications on board at that time, but because they had so many unmediated psychotic episodes, their brain is literally damaged and doesn't respond to the medications. Mania episodes are known for their high levels of glutamate (excitatory brain chemical). High glutamate is very toxic to the brain, and the brain begins to get worse and worse with each mania episode. Medications help the brain not get into these states in the first place, thus preserving the brain from further damage. Newer antidepressants and newer antipsychotics actually increase a special protein in your brain called Brain-Derived Neurotrophic Factor (BDNF). BDNF is a protein that helps your brain create new connections and help protect the brain from damage. So not only do these medications help prevent damage, but it also contributes to creating new brain connections and guarding the brain against damage.

Are there legitimate reasons for being scared of medications or not wanting to take them? Absolutely! They do have side effects that can occur (keyword is *can*, not *will*), and, yes, some medications can make you feel sedated. Some can raise your risk of weight gain, diabetes, and high cholesterol! I can understand why people don't want to take medications. The decision to take medications will be based on a benefit vs. risk ratio. This assessment isn't anything new. We do benefit vs. risk ratios all the time in life. Do I enjoy this cake at the risk of adding unwanted weight? Do I drive a car fast to get to my job at the risk of getting into a car accident? The same goes for treatment, and especially medications. For some, the benefits of medications are as clear as day, for others, it may be a mishmash of feeling better here, but feeling worse here and not there. Finding the right medication and what combinations, if any, works for you takes time and frustration. The good news is that new medications that come out have fewer side effects. We are moving to a place where we can also pinpoint which medications will work the first time through gene assessment. Just for now (in 2019), we are stuck with some trial and error, just like finding that blood pressure medication that does its job but doesn't give you side effects.

And then there is the opposite position. Medications are viewed as "cure-alls." If there is an issue, the pill will take care of it. This, too, is not realistic with psychiatric medications. Can psychiatric medications help you with tough emotions and moods (and psychosis)? Yes, but that doesn't take away the root causes of depression or anxiety. An example I use is diet and exercise. Say you eat 3000 calories of pure sugar and fatty foods daily. You start to gain unwanted weight and feel depressed about this. You learn that exercise can help with your unwanted weight issue, so you start working out. You are not happy with working out because you get sore, feel exhausted afterward, but you make some progress with desired weight loss. You are still eating the same 3000 calorie diet, but the exercise is helping. Here the exercise is medications. Sure, exercise is helping manage the weight gain, but the root cause is the high-calorie unhealthy diet.

The high-calorie diet can represent a lot of things: past trauma, shame, guilt, sadness, inadequacy, poor self-esteem, hopelessness, anxiety, panic, and more. It's not that exercise is useless, it's just managing the weight gain, just like medications manage depression or anxiety. But getting to the core, the driving factors are key. Say this person maintained a 2000 calorie diet or plant-based foods AND exercised? Well, they would benefit greatly. This is why medications are helpful and an important part of treatment, but they will never be a "cure-all." The combination of different types of treatments is an all-around best scenario for anyone with mental illness.

Primer on brain function (neurons/synapses), structures

This section is a basic introduction to brain structures and brain function related to mental health. You don't, by all means, have to read this section to understand how medications and treatment work in mental health. This is more of a "for your information."

The brain is the most complex and intricate organ we have. There are approximately 100 billion neurons in the brain. Neurons are little phone lines that connect to tell parts of the brain to do certain things. Neurons "fire" all the time. Right now, as you read this, neurons are firing to allow you to see, allow you to comprehend writing, find meaning in the text, maintain your breathing, keep your organs functioning optimally, and so much more. Neurons "talk" to each other by chemicals. These chemicals tell the receiving neuron what to do and how to tell the next neuron. A way to see this is to imagine you can communicate via writing to people. You (a neuron) write a letter with instructions (chemical) and then pass it along to another person (another neuron), who then reads those instructions and then gives written instructions to the next person and so on. These chemicals in the brain are called neurotransmitters. There are many types of neurotransmitters, and we have discussed a lot of them in the book already. Each neurotransmitter has its own instructions that are unique to itself. This is why we target certain neurotransmitters over others. Neurotransmitters need to be in a balance to be optimal. Too little and the neurons don't "fire" as much, too much, and they "fire" too much. We are born with certain wiring from our parents. We have luck with some balanced neurotransmitters, but we also have unbalanced neurotransmitters. Depending on the type of neurotransmitter and the severity of the unbalance is where we start to see if mental conditions form will express themselves.

The brain is like a muscle. You exercise certain areas; they become stronger, you don't exercise certain areas, they become weaker. This is for our benefit typically because it creates efficiency. There is no point in having strong neuron structures for the sucking reflex seen in infants when you are 44 years old. We use the term, "if it fires, it wires." This is important to know because the more symptoms of mental illness, like anxiety and depression, persist, the more hardwired and resistant they become. This is why you can meet someone who has had untreated depression for 30 years who literally cannot or has great difficulty picking up on positive events. Traumatic responses work this way too. You experience a terrifying event, and your brain's alarm system becomes very strong. It then dominates, leaving the part of the brain that helps regulate emotions to get weaker and weaker. This is why psychotherapy works. You start to practice the new thoughts, the new coping skills, the new perspectives, and your brain starts to fire in those areas that have been weakened and starts to strengthen them. So yes, psychotherapy can transform your brain (and for the better!).

Brain Structures Worth Knowing

Prefrontal Cortex (sometimes called the neocortex) - this is the newest addition to the human brain. Located right behind your forehead, the prefrontal cortex helps you make decisions and control impulses. Controlling and moderating emotions is also a part of the prefrontal cortex's job. Socializing and being able to connect with others is a core feature of the prefrontal cortex and is partially what makes us social beings, along with the benefits of working together and delayed gratification.

Limbic System - this is our old primal part of the brain. This is your emotional and fear center. It also helps with memory, learning, and motivation. The infamous fight or flight is located in this part of the brain. The goal of the limbic system is survival (fight or flight, learning, motivation) and reproduction (lust). Anxiety, agitation, anger, sadness, panic, lust, and impulsive behaviors are located here. Sometimes you will hear of the word "amygdala," which is purely emotional senses. It is a part of the limbic system. Hippocampus is also located within the limbic system and is important in new memory formation. This is important because the brain wants to learn from scary experiences (fright, panic, anxiety) to prevent these from happening again. When the limbic system isn't working properly, odd things happen to the hippocampus and your memories. Say you have depression, and your limbic system is sad. Remembering new information may be very hard and remembering past events will be hued by the depression. So literally, it is harder for depressed people to remember positive events in their lives. Extreme trauma and agitation can lead to the hippocampus switching off or fragmenting memory formation. In PTSD or trauma events (such as rape), remembering details of the traumatic event can be very difficult. It is your brain's way of "giving you a break" from the horrendous nature just experienced. The only problem is that the body picks up on that trauma and the trauma comes out in all these odd ways that we see in PTSD. Part of PTSD treatment is going over the story over and over to reconfigure the memory so that your body can learn that the trauma had a beginning and an end and move on from the trauma.

Antidepressant

Selective Serotonin Reuptake Inhibitors (SSRI)

Medication names: fluoxetine (Prozac), citalopram (Celexa), escitalopram (Lexapro), sertraline (Zoloft), paroxetine (Paxil), fluvoxamine (Luvox)

How does it work?

SSRIs are a very common antidepressant that can also work for anxiety. They are considered to be first-line treatment for depression and anxiety disorders. SSRI's work by increasing the amount of the brain chemical serotonin, which helps with feeling well, impulse control, sleep, and appetite. Normally, when serotonin is released from one neuron to another, there is a vacuum cleaner that sucks up excess serotonin and recycles it back into the first neuron so that it may be used again. SSRIs stop these vacuum cleaners, which leaves more serotonin to hit the next neuron. When the next neuron gets more serotonin, it fires more in the parts of the brain that help you feel well, and this can help uplift you out of depression and also help alleviate anxiety.

How long does it take to work, and what should I expect?

SSRI's can take upwards of 4-8 weeks to reach full effect. Some people (called super-responders) can start to feel better within 2-5 days. SSRI's are sometimes misunderstood as medications because of poor education from the prescriber. Many people do not know that it can take that long, so after 2-3 days, they stop it because they are expecting an effect quickly. SSRIs usually take longer than other medications to have any effect. As stated above, SSRI's leave more serotonin for the next neuron to fire. That neuron accepting serotonin uses "tunnels" to allow the serotonin into the neuron.

I liken this to the drain in your shower. Typically, you only need one drain to accept the shower water without any issues. If you start to flood the shower tub with water, that one drain is going to have difficulty accepting all that water. So, you have to build more drains in the tub in order to take in that water efficiently. That's what happens in the brain. The increase in serotonin cannot be accepted right away because there are too few tunnels. They haven't needed anymore because it has been used to this low level of serotonin. Now, with more serotonin, the receiving neuron learns it needs to build more tunnels in order to take the extra serotonin. To build these tunnels in the receiving neuron takes about 4-8 weeks, and that's why SSRIs can take that long to have full effect. Think of your brain as having a "under construction" sign on each neuron as they build more tunnels to take in the extra serotonin.

Typically, SSRIs have a gradual effect. Feeling fully better won't happen overnight but in a more subtle matter. This can make it hard to determine if the SSRI is working or not as the effects are very gradual. There are sometimes that an SSRI can actually make you more anxious for the first few weeks. This is due to the brain trying to regulate the new serotonin fluctuations. This almost always dissipates, and most people ride it out, although if it is impairing and very uncomfortable, you will want to call the prescriber right away. Typically, after the trial period, if the SSRI has had a partial effect (taking away some symptoms), then an increase in the dosage will most likely occur. If, after the trial period, there is no effect or has intolerable side effects, then the SSRI could be switched out for another antidepressant by the prescriber.

Specific Differences

Prozac (fluoxetine) - Prozac is the first SSRI created back in 1987. Prozac is known for its "energizing" effect, which can be useful in depression that exhibits low motivation, poor energy, and increased sleepiness. Prozac also has a very long half-life, which is a fancy talk for "Prozac lasts a long time in your body." This can be good for people who frequently miss taking their medication daily as they will tend to have some coverage from the previous pill.

Paxil (paroxetine) and **Luvox (fluvoxamine)** - Both Paxil and Luvox are both known to be more on the sedating side. This can be good for people with sleep insomnia or high anxiety, as it can help cool the fires of anxiety. Luvox is very well known to be a good SSRI for OCD, but Luvox is very underutilized due to its cross interactions with many different types of medications.

Zoloft (sertraline) - Zoloft, like Prozac, can have some energizing features to it. Zoloft is FDA approved for PTSD and is seen very frequently in the VA health system. Of all the SSRIs, Zoloft is the least likely to have any weight gain and can actually help some people lose weight. This can be a good or bad thing, depending on you.

Celexa (citalopram) and **Lexapro (escitalopram)** - I consider both Celexa and Lexapro to be "middle line" SSRIs. Generally, they are right in the middle of being not sedating, but not energizing and not gaining weight but not losing weight. Celexa at high dosages (60mg or above) can cause some heart rhythm issues in people prone to heart issues, so generally, the dosage will max out at 40mg. Lexapro is chemically similar to Celexa but is broken down one step further. This is nice because Lexapro doesn't have the heart issue that Celexa has. There are some studies that show that Lexapro may be the fastest acting SSRI on the market.

Side Effects

Because SSRIs deal with serotonin, and serotonin is a regulator of appetite, nausea can occur and is the most frequent side effect. As with most side effects to medications, these tend to dissipate over time. Headache can also be a frequent side effect experienced, but again, tends to wear off by the end of month one or two. The number one reason people stop an SSRI is because of the side effect of sexual dysfunction. Although side effects don't always happen, when sexual dysfunction occurs due to SSRI, it can cause a lot of personal challenges for the person taking it. Men may have trouble with erections. Women may have decreased libido. Both men and women may have trouble reaching orgasm. And unlike other side effects, sexual dysfunction with SSRIs tends to persist over time. What can be done if you have sexual dysfunction on an SSRI? You can switch to another antidepressant that has no sexual side effects (most common is Wellbutrin and Remeron) or add Wellbutrin to get more antidepressant coverage along with mitigating the sexual side effect.

Serotonin Syndrome
Serotonin Syndrome can be remembered by the mnemonic **HARMFUL**
Hyperthermia - high fever
Anti Cognitive - delirium, confusion
Reflexes - easily startled reflexes, highly sensitive reflexes
Myoclonus - jerking and twitching
Fast Heart Rate - above 100 beats per minute
Unconsciousness - loss of consciousness can occur
Loss of Urine, Diarrhea - loss of control of bladder and digestive system

Table 3.1 Serotonin Syndrome Signs and Symptoms

SSRIs can cause some anxiety and difficulty sleeping at the beginning of use. This seems counterintuitive as a lot of people take an SSRI for anxiety, but the way regulation takes part in the brain can sometimes increase anxiety. This tends to go away after 1-2 months. Weight gain and sedation tend to be unusual with SSRIs, but some people do report weight gain from certain SSRIs, so I tend not to negate it. In very rare cases, adverse effects can happen with SSRIs, such as low sodium levels, rare seizures, and serotonin syndrome.

Black Box Warning

Many antidepressants have a "black box warning" on the medication, which is an FDA requirement is there is a part of the medication that can be a "serious hazard". The "black box warning" on anti-depressants states that young adults (ages 18-24) can develop increased suicidal thoughts and suicide attempts. This seems counter-intuitive due to the antidepressants supposedly trying to help reduce suicidal thoughts. There are certain explanations to this, but none are certain. Some include that antidepressants can sometimes put an "undiagnosed bipolar" into a mania episode. This means that a person who is being treated for major depression might really have bipolar but have never had a manic episode. With depression and suicidal thoughts, the person then becomes more energetic, more impulsive, but the suicidal thoughts remain and haven't been helped by the medication yet. This can lead to an increase in suicide attempts. Most results from multiple studies state that anti-depressants raise the suicide attempt rate from 2% to 4% of the young population who take anti-depressants. Compare this to the 15% suicide attempt rate of untreated depression and the other major risks with untreated depression.

Mental Conditions Used For: depressive disorders, anxiety disorders, trauma and PTSD, bipolar, impulse control issues, eating disorders

Serotonin-Norepinephrine Reuptake Inhibitor (SNRI)

Medication names: venlafaxine (Effexor), desvenlafaxine (Pristiq), duloxetine (Cymbalta)

How does it work?

SNRIs work very similarly to SSRIs. The main difference between the two is what brain chemicals they target. While SSRIs target serotonin, SNRI target serotonin and norepinephrine. SNRIs work by increasing the amount of the brain chemicals serotonin and norepinephrine, which helps with feeling well, impulse control, sleep, and appetite, as well as norepinephrine effects of increased energy, motivation, and concentration. Normally, when one of these brain chemicals are released from one neuron to another, there is a vacuum cleaner that sucks up excess serotonin and recycles it back into the first neuron so that it may be used again. SNRIs stop these vacuum cleaners, which leaves more of the targeted brain chemicals to hit the next neuron. When the next neuron gets more serotonin or norepinephrine, it fires more in the parts of the brain that help you feel well, and this can help uplift you out of depression and also help alleviate anxiety. SNRIs, especially Cymbalta, can help alleviate chronic neuropathic pain. This is the type of pain typically of a nerve origin, so think numb, tingles, sharp, lightning, pinched nerves, etc.. This can be an added benefit as many people with depression have co-occurring pain disorders.

How long does it take to work, and what should I expect?

Like SSRIs, SNRIs can take upwards of 4-8 weeks to reach full efficacy. This is due to the "construction" the brain has to do in order to accept the new amount of serotonin and norepinephrine. Also, like SSRIs, the effects tend to creep in rather than have a very noticeable effect. These are not like a pain pill or anxiety pill that gets immediate relief, but by week 2-4, you should be able to notice improvements in mood, less irritability, reduced anxiety, and whatever else it is targeting. SNRIs can be activating initially - meaning that they can cause some anxiety and restlessness. This tends to wear off with time. Given it can take 4-8 weeks to see if the medication will work well or not, if side effects occur and are unbearable, you will want to inform your prescriber as soon as possible.

Specific Differences

Effexor (venlafaxine) - Effexor is one of the most well-known SNRIs. Effexor is funny because it seems to be more like an SSRI (only increasing serotonin) in the low-mid range dosing and then becomes an SNRI when increased passed 225mg, although this may vary with some people. Effexor is very well known for its withdrawal symptoms (increased anxiety and depression) if it is stopped right away. If you want to stop Effexor, you should call the prescriber and have them taper the medication to avoid such withdrawals.

Pristiq (desvenlafaxine)- the odd cousin of Effexor (venlafaxine), Pristiq is not readily seen in practice. There really isn't any particular reason for this as far as I know. Pristiq is different than Effexor because of Pristiq's ability to increase a little more norepinephrine than Effexor. Like Effexor, Pristiq has nasty withdrawal if stopped abruptly. It should be tapered by your prescriber to avoid such withdrawal symptoms.

Cymbalta (duloxetine) - the sexier cousin of Effexor and Pristiq, Cymbalta has the known properties of an SNRI but also is well established as an SNRI that helps with pain, specifically fatigue, nerve pain, and somatic pain. Cymbalta is FDA approved for fibromyalgia, diabetic neuropathic pain, and chronic musculoskeletal pain. Since depression can present with pain symptoms or someone can be depressed because of pain, Cymbalta offers hope to help relieve depression, anxiety, and nasty pain symptoms.

Side Effects

SNRIs are very similar to SSRIs with the addition of boosting norepinephrine. Because SNRIs deal with serotonin, and serotonin is a regulator of appetite, nausea can occur and is the most frequent side effect. With norepinephrine, you can typically get some anxiety and restlessness. As with most side effects to medications, these tend to dissipate over time. Headache can also be a frequent side effect experienced. The number one reason people stop an SNRI is because of the side effect of sexual dysfunction. Men may have trouble with erections. Women may have decreased libido. Both men and women may have trouble reaching orgasm. And like SSRIs, sexual dysfunction with SNRIs tends to persist over time. What can be done if you have sexual dysfunction on an SNRI? You can switch to another antidepressant that has no sexual side effects (most common is Wellbutrin and Remeron) or add Wellbutrin to get more antidepressant coverage along with mitigating the sexual side effect. SNRIs can cause some anxiety and difficulty sleeping in the beginning of use. This seems counterintuitive as a lot of people take an SNRI for anxiety, but the way regulation takes part in the brain can sometimes increase anxiety. This tends to go away after 1-2 months. Weight gain and sedation tend to be unusual with SNRIs. In very rare cases, adverse effects can happen with SNRIs, such as low sodium levels, rare seizures, and serotonin syndrome.

Mental Conditions Used for: depressive disorders, anxiety disorders, trauma and PTSD, bipolar, impulse control issues, eating disorders, chronic pain

Norepinephrine-Dopamine Reuptake Inhibitor (NDRI)

Medication names: bupropion (Wellbutrin)

How does it work?

NDRIs are a relatively newer type of antidepressant. The only NDRI is bupropion, or brand name Wellbutrin. NDRIs were created for depression that doesn't respond to serotonin. NDRIs target the brain chemicals dopamine and norepinephrine. Dopamine helps us with pleasure, motivation, and learning. Norepinephrine, as we learned from SNRIs, helps with concentration, energy, focus, and motivation. NDRIs work the same as SSRIs and SNRIs. They turn off the "vacuums" that suck up extra norepinephrine and dopamine between each brain cell (or neuron). This leads to more norepinephrine and dopamine being available to activate the next neuron and increase firing in areas related to mood.

How long does it take to work, and what should I expect?

The average time to reach full effectiveness is 4-8 weeks, much like other antidepressants. This is due to the neuron needing to construct new "drains" to allow the new high amount of norepinephrine and dopamine into the neurons. Wellbutrin is known for its "energizing effects," which can be liberating for some and terrifying for others due to perceived anxiety. No matter the case, the spike in energy does tend to regulate out within a month or two. Increased anxiety is the number one reason why people stop NDRIs, so if it is intolerable, then simply call your prescriber.

Specific Difference

As of now (2019), bupropion is the only NDRI on the market. NDRIs are very useful for the type of depression that results in low motivation, poor energy, poor focus, too much sleep, eating too much, and no pleasure in pleasurable activities. NDRIs don't work as well for agitated-type depression. They have been shown to be helpful with generalized anxiety, but not for panic attacks as the increased stimulation can trigger more panic attacks. Also, know that NDRIs are commonly added to SSRIs or SNRIs to get boosts of serotonin, norepinephrine, and dopamine for optimal depression relief. One of the big benefits of NDRIs over other antidepressants is that there are no sexual side effects. Another known benefit is that NDRIs can be used to help someone stop nicotine. This is due to NDRIs increase in norepinephrine, which is the same brain chemical raised by nicotine.

Side Effects

The side effects of NDRIs are different than SSRIs and SNRIs as they target different brain chemicals. As stated above, increased energy and anxiety are a very common side effect, at least initially. The increased energy can put some people on edge and feel impulsive and anxious. This typically levels out although, if it is too uncomfortable or interfering with daily life, it is time to call your prescriber. NDRIs can cause some "drying effects," like dry mouth, constipation, and also some nausea. Because of the potential energy activation, insomnia and headache can occur as well. Sweating, low appetite (weight loss), along with raises in blood pressure, can also occur with NDRIs. Adverse effects can generally be avoided but include seizures (higher risk if they are abusing alcohol or benzodiazepines) and inducing a manic episode if the person has undiagnosed bipolar disorder.

Mental Conditions Used for: major depressive disorder, seasonal affective disorder, nicotine addiction, ADHD, and sexual dysfunction

Tricyclic Antidepressant (TCA)

Medication names: amitriptyline (Elavil), amoxapine (Asendin), clomipramine (Anafranil), desipramine (Norpramin), dothiepin (Prothiaden), doxepin (Sinequan), imipramine (Tofranil), lofepramine (Deprimyl), maprotiline (Ludiomil), nortriptyline (Pamelor), protriptyline (Tristan), trimipramine (Surmontil)

How does it work?

TCAs are not called "Tri" because they work on 3 brain chemicals. Rather, it is named "tri" because the molecule has three atoms. TCAs were one of the first antidepressants in the markets. TCAs work by blocking the pumps that suck back up the brain chemicals serotonin and norepinephrine. This leads to increases of serotonin and norepinephrine in the brain, which will help increase feelings of well-being (serotonin), reduce anxiety (serotonin), and increase energy and concentration (norepinephrine). Theoretically, there is some dopamine action in TCAs, but none at a level that we appreciate. Because norepinephrine is increased, chronic pain, especially nerve pain, can be relieved with TCAs. TCAs are not seen as much anymore because of the advent of SSRIs and SNRIs, which have far fewer side effects and target more precisely the areas we want increases in.

How long does it take to work, and what should I expect?

Like SSRIs and SNRIs, TCAs can take upwards of 2-6 weeks to be effective for depression. It may be more immediate for anxiety and insomnia as TCAs can have some sedation. Generally, if you are being started on a TCA, you have tried other antidepressants as TCAs are not typically first-line treatment. Expectations should be slow increases in wellbeing and less negativity. TCAs are not like a benzodiazepine like Valium or Xanax that has a punch. The effects will be gradual but will get there.

Specific Differences

There are many TCAs in the market. Simply going through each one would not be advantageous as many are not relatively used anymore. Instead, we will focus on the most commonly seen TCAs in the mental health field.

Doxepin (Sinequan) - doxepin is a commonly used TCA for both depression, anxiety, but especially seen used for insomnia. The dosages for insomnia tend to be considerably less than the antidepressant dosages, so side effects are generally less.

Amitriptyline (Elavil) - amitriptyline is a very common TCA used for pain control. Before the induction of Cymbalta and Lyrica, amitriptyline was the main go-to for nerve pain, most commonly Fibromyalgia. Today it is still used for these issues. You will also see amitriptyline used in depression and anxiety, especially OCD.

Clomipramine (Anafranil) - this common TCA is used quite frequently in OCD. Clomipramine at the highest dosages is one of two medications have the best evidence to help with OCD

Side Effects

TCAs are known for their side effects, unfortunately. They are very strong "anticholinergics," which is known to "dry you out." Drying out refers to dry mouth, blurry vision, constipation, urinary retention (not urinating), and in more severe cases, delirium. TCAs can cause emotional flattening, likened to the "zombie effect," which includes sedation and drowsiness. TCAs can cause the normal gamete of serotonin-related side effects, such as nausea, vomiting, and headache. In more rare cases but needs to be considered, TCAs can cause heart issues such as rhythm disturbances, low blood pressure, and high heart rate. Because of these side effects, TCAs can be very dangerous to someone who overdoses on them. A thorough assessment should always include how suicidal a person is before giving a TCA because they are very lethal if overdosed on. Like most side effects, most dissipate with time, and the medication becomes more adjusted, but you can see why we use TCAs are second-line medications as the side effect profile is large and impairing for some.

Mental Conditions Used for: depressive disorders (especially treatment-resistant depression), anxiety disorders (especially obsessive compulsive disorder), insomnia, and pain (such as Fibromyalgia)

Monoamine Oxidase Inhibitor (MAOi)

Medication names: isocarboxazid (Marplan), phenelzine (Nardil), tranylcypromine (Parnate), nialamide (Niamid), selegiline (Deprenyl), safinamide (Xadago), phenoxypropazine (Drazine), safrazine (Safra), minaprine (Cantor), and many more that are very rarely seen or used

How does it work?

The MAOi's glory days were the 1950s - 1970s. They were considered the first depressant targeted medication. MAOi's work by stopping the enzyme that breaks down "monoamines," which are a certain type of neurotransmitter. The target neurotransmitters that were the focus of MAOi medications were serotonin, epinephrine, melatonin, and dopamine. The problem with MAOi's is that they are not that selective. They end up inadvertently increasing many other neurotransmitters in the brain, which can cause havoc. The most notorious and well known for MAOi's is that of tyramine, which is normally broken down by enzymes. MAOi's don't allow these important enzymes to break down tyramine, which can lead to tyramine increasing to dangerous levels. These dangerous levels of tyramine lead to extremely high levels of norepinephrine, which then can lead to extremely high blood pressure. This dangerous high blood pressure can lead to damage to organs and unexpectedly cause heart issues, such as heart attacks as well as strokes. Avoiding foods with tyramine is an essential with MAOi's. These foods include aged cheese, wine, beer, fermented foods (kimchi, sour cream, yogurt), pickled foods, soy sauce, chocolate, and processed deli meats. Good luck with those restrictions

How long does it take to work and what should I expect?

MAOi medications are rarely used anymore. If you have a person on an MAOi, they have generally been on it for many years and it's the ONLY antidepressant that works for them. IF there is a new start with an MAOi, there better be very good rationales for such initiations, such as treatment resistance and trials with all the other types of antidepressants. Generally speaking, if you start a MAOi, you can expect to see results in 2-4 weeks. Help with insomnia can be immediate.

Specific Differences

As MAOi's are rarely, if ever used, the specific differences are minimal and not particularly worth investing your time into reading. Most likely, if you or a family member are experiencing MAOi's in your life, they have been used for many years and are familiar.

Side Effects

MAOi's are notorious for their side effects. These were, indeed, the very first antidepressants, so we are talking about research that is now almost 70 years old. MAOi's, as stated above, have a huge reaction with foods that contain tyramine. Those foods are listed above in the "how it works" section. MAOi's are well known for their interactions with other medications. These interactions can lead to very uncomfortable side effects and adverse effects. The most common side effects are dizziness, headaches, sedation, tremors, weakness, blurring vision, dry mouth, constipation, and sexual dysfunction. You will also see nausea and increased sweating. More severe adverse effects include seizures, high blood pressure crisis, and liver damage.

Mental Conditions Used for: depressive disorders, anxiety disorders

Other Anti-Depressants

Medication names: mirtazapine (Remeron), nefazodone (Serzone), trazodone (Desyrel), vilazodone (Viibryd), vortioxetine (Trintellix, formerly Brintellix)

How does it work?

Mirtazapine (Remeron) - classified as noradrenaline and specific serotonergic agent (NaSSA), mirtazapine is a unique antidepressant that is very commonly seen. It works by blocking a different type of receptor called the alpha receptor. Blocking this alpha receptor increases both norepinephrine and serotonin in the brain, which helps with anxiety and depression. Mirtazapine also blocks histamine, a brain chemical that is key in allergic reactions but also creates arousal of your body's system. Blocking histamine makes your sedated, which is why mirtazapine is a great sleep aid.

Nefazodone (Serzone) - not commonly seen, nefazodone is a serotonin antagonist reuptake inhibitor(SARI). These work by blocking the pumps that suck up serotonin, which leaves more serotonin in the brain to help alleviate depression and anxiety.

Trazodone (Desyrel)- another serotonin antagonist reuptake inhibitor (SARI), trazodone works by blocking the pumps that suck up serotonin. Trazodone is very well known for its sedation rather than a good antidepressant. You will typically see trazodone used for insomnia more than an antidepressant.

Vilazodone (Viibryd) - the newest of the new (in 2019). Vilazodone is a serotonin partial agonist reuptake inhibitor (SPARI). It works by, again, blocking the pumps that suck up serotonin. The main difference with vilazodone is that it has this "partial agonist" feature. What this in simple terms means is that it allows just a little bit of serotonin not to be sucked up. What does this do? Theoretically, it lessens the sexual side effects of many antidepressants, which is the number one reason why people stop antidepressants.

Vortioxetine (Trintellix) - another newest of the new (in 2019). Vortioxetine is a serotonin multimodal (S-MM). What on earth does that mean? It works on a whole slew of brain chemicals (making it "multi"). It releases (increases) serotonin (feeling well-being), norepinephrine (energy, concentration), dopamine (pleasure and motivation), glutamate (energy), acetylcholine (focus, concentration), and histamine (energy). As you can see, this medication targets many different brain chemicals than we normally target, which makes this medication a very specific medication for specific type of depression. Read the specific differences to see the purpose of this antidepressant.

How long does it take to work, and what should I expect?

Mirtazapine (Remeron) - mirtazapine, like other serotonin antidepressants, takes about 4-6 weeks to see any effect. The effects will be gradual and will work slowly. The sleeping part of mirtazapine should be like a sleep agent and work within 30 minutes of taking. That being said, if it doesn't work well as a sleep aid the first night, try it for at least another 3-4 nights before deciding to switch it out.

Nefazodone (Serzone) - nefazodone takes around 2-6 weeks to start noticing effects for depression. Because nefazodone is sedating, use for sleep and anxiety should be rather immediate (within 30 minutes of taking medication).

The effects of depression will be gradual.

Trazodone (Desyrel) - trazodone is almost solely used for sleep. For sleep, you should know if it is working for you after about 2-3 nights of usage. You should start feeling tired about 30 - 60 minutes after taking the medication.

Vilazodone (Viibryd) - considered to be one of the fastest-acting antidepressants, vilazodone can start working after one week. The full effect will generally not be reached until 4-6 weeks later, though, so remain taking the medication for that time to see if the medication is a good fit.

Vortioxetine (Trintellix) - you may start to feel better on vortioxetine between weeks 2-4. Such feelings will be gradual and slow. Always wait the full 6-8 weeks of trying vortioxetine to see if it'll work for you.

Specific Differences

Mirtazapine (Remeron) - mirtazapine is a well-known antidepressant. It is known to be a good medication for depression, anxiety, and insomnia, and appetite stimulator. Frequently, you'll see mirtazapine used in post-traumatic stress disorder (PTSD), as it works well with agitation and anxiety seen in PTSD along with sleep disturbances. Mirtazapine is a good medication for elderly people as it tends to not have a lot of cross interactions with other medications. Another great feature of mirtazapine is that it generally has no sexual side effects.

Nefazodone (Serzone) - not a very common antidepressant but still seen in the mental health field. Nefazodone is typically used in treatment-resistant depression, or depression that has been trialed on many medications with no relief. It can be used for anxiety as well but not as common. It is generally used as a last line of medications because it is known for potentially causing liver damage.

Trazodone (Desyrel) - not a spectacular antidepressant medication, but a great sleep agent. Trazodone is a good sleep aid that generally is tolerated very well by many people. There is little risk of dependence and tolerance (having to have it/needing more to get the same effect) with trazodone compared to other sleep medications like Ambien or Lunesta. The dosages for sleep are generally much lower than for antidepressant treatment. Generally, you'll see trazodone being used between 50mg and 200mg for sleep and 150mg to 375mg for depression.

Vilazodone (Viibryd) - being one of the newer antidepressants, we get excited because it's new and maybe the next best thing, but at the same time, we don't have enough data to know its effects long term. Vilazodone's claim to fame is being an antidepressant that works as an SSRI but has less chance of sexual side effects. Studies show that there is, indeed, less sexual side effects with Vilazodone than with SSRIs and SNRIs, but state that there are still some sexual side effects with Vilazodone. Personally, this is not a medication I have prescribed much at this moment in time so my personal and anecdotal knowledge of how it is with sexual side effects with patients is essentially null.

Vortioxetine (Trintellix) - Vortioxetine is also a newer antidepressant on the market. It's claim to fame is that it is highly selective at certain receptors in the brain. Saving you from the complications of this medication, it seems to be a good antidepressant for depression that has cognitive issues. These cognitive issues include poor memory, decision making, "fog," forgetfulness, and difficulty thinking. This tends to be in depression that is more of the "slowing" type depression, rather than the more anxious type depression. It actually is not a good selection for anxiety, not only because it may not treat it, but it may also make it worse. There are studies that show that that Vortioxetine has fewer sexual side effects than more traditional SSRIs and SNRIs.

Side Effects

Mirtazapine (Remeron) - mirtazapine is known for its sedation (drowsiness) and weight gain. These can be great side effects for a person who is not sleeping or is not eating enough. It can be detrimental if you are always tired or overweight. Mirtazapine has a strong "anticholinergic" effect meaning it "dries" you out. This drying is dry mouth, urinary retention (holding urine), and constipation. Mirtazapine can also cause dizziness and low blood pressure

Nefazodone (Serzone) - nefazodone is a known "anticholinergic," causing dry mouth, constipation, and urinary retention. It can also cause increased appetite (weight gain) and sedation. Of course, nefazodone is known for its liver damage and, thus, used as a last resort medication

Trazodone (Desyrel) - trazodone is well known for its sedation. This is a good thing as we use it for sleep. The side effects we don't like are nausea, blurred vision, constipation, dry mouth, headache, and dizziness. Trazodone is colloquially called "trazo-bone," and this is because trazodone is known for a rare side effect called priapism. This is a painful long-lasting erection that is a medical emergency and of course, comes with added embarrassment.

Vilazodone (Viibryd) - vilazodone can cause nausea, diarrhea, vomiting, and dry mouth. Interestingly enough, some people still get sexual side effects, although lower than traditional SSRIs and SNRIs. Insomnia and dizziness can also occur

Vortioxetine (Trintellix) - vortioxetine has some of the lowest side effects of any antidepressant. Generally, nausea, constipation, and sexual dysfunction are the main side effects. Even then, the sexual side effects occur at a much lower prevalence compared to traditional SSRIs and SNRIs.

Mental Conditions Used For: Depressive Disorders, Anxiety Disorders, PTSD, Insomnia

Anti-anxiety

Benzodiazepines

Medication names: lorazepam (Ativan), alprazolam (Xanax), clonazepam (Klonopin), diazepam (Valium), chlordiazepoxide (Librium), oxazepam (Serax)

How does it work?

Benzodiazepines work well. VERY well. They work by increasing the main chemical that helps us remain calm, which is GABA. When you take a benzodiazepine, this increase in GABA is not only calming, but benzodiazepines also slow down the rapid-fire in the amygdala, which is your fear center. There are many different types of GABA receptors, but the GABA-A receptor is where benzodiazepines hit. GABA-A is the receptor you want to hit if you want a powerful punch. This is the same receptor that alcohol attaches too, hence why you get drunk. The problem is that the GABA-A receptor is very volatile and erratic. It's effects can cause big swings up and down, along with build tolerance (needing more benzo to get the same effect) and dependence (needing the medication or else feeling worse. This is why benzodiazepines are typically used only for short term, if used at all. Once you get someone started, stopping them can mean really bad rebound anxiety, to the point that they are worse than when they started. Because of the big punch that benzodiazepines give at the GABA-A site, benzodiazepines are readily sought after to abuse.

How long does it take to work, and what should I expect?

One of the benefits of benzodiazepines is that they are quick acting. Within 15-30 minutes after taking a benzodiazepine, your anxiety will melt away for the most part. This is, in part, why people like them so much. To have a medication that can alleviate the anxiety that quickly and effectively is very powerful. If you are taking a benzodiazepine for the first time, always take it in a safe environment and do not operate any machines (car, lawnmower, etc.) as these can be very sedating. You always want to watch out for how much you are taking. If you find yourself taking more and more to get the same effect, this is not a good sign and will only get worse unless you taper off the benzodiazepines. Like I stated before: short term and for emergencies only. Unfortunately, I see prescribers give benzodiazepines out very readily and for odd reasons. Lorazepam 1mg at bedtime for sleep for instance. That medication is ordered to be taken every night for how long? Indefinitely? If so, then that person will need increases in the dosages to keep the same effect over that time along with having terrible insomnia if stopping the benzodiazepine. This doesn't even consider the research on long term benzodiazepine use causing cognitive and memory issues later in life. Soon you may see this person needing 4-6mg at bedtime to get the same effect. Stopping the medication abruptly can cause seizures and even death. Don't ever stop a benzodiazepine on your own. The risks are too high. Talk to your prescriber and taper the dosages down.

Specific Differences

All benzodiazepines work the same way. The main differences between the different types of benzodiazepines are the intensity and how long they last

Diazepam (Valium) - generally a long-lasting benzodiazepine, often seen in panic disorder and very often in alcohol/benzodiazepine detoxification. It does still have a risk though.

Clonazepam (Klonopin) - a long-lasting benzodiazepine generally seen as the "safer" option than other benzodiazepines. Please note that there is still a risk for dependency and tolerance building from clonazepam

Alprazolam (Xanax) - by far, one of the most powerful and fastest to leave the body, often leaving the person wanting more. Very high risk for dependence and tolerance with alprazolam and very often sought out in the black market

Lorazepam (Ativan) - fast-moderate acting benzodiazepine. Tends to be more predictable than alprazolam and very often seen in alcohol/benzodiazepine detoxification

Side Effects

Sedation is the main side effect to be on the alert for. People do drive cars or do other activities that can be very detrimental to their and others' well-being. Remember, if you are under the influence of benzodiazepines (even if prescribed) and you get into an accident or pulled over, you may be tested for sobriety. If you fail, it's treated the same as drunk driving. Fatigue, worsening depression, and dizziness are very common side effects. Memory issues and confusion can be a side effect, and long term use can cause permanent memory and cognitive loss. Adverse effects include taking too many and having your breathing slow or stop, leading to death.

Mental Conditions Used For: anxiety disorders (especially panic disorder), seizure prevention or active seizures, insomnia (although should not be used for insomnia), agitation/violence

Buspirone (Buspar)

How does it work?

Buspirone was initially created and marketed as an antipsychotic in 1975. As further studies of the medication went further, they learned that it really didn't do anything for psychosis. Instead, they discovered it actually was affecting a whole other receptor than what they were going for. That receptor, 5-HT1A, is a major serotonin receptor that helps calm our body. And with that, the buspirone was approved for use in generalized anxiety. By attaching to the 5-HT1A site, the brain decreases norepinephrine (excitatory brain chemical), while also increasing serotonin (calming, well-being brain chemical) in the brain.

How long does it take to work, and what should I expect?

In general, buspirone takes about 2-4 weeks to reach efficacy and to know whether the medication will work for you. Buspirone is a funny medication. For some, it is godsent, relieving most of their generalized anxiety. For others, it might as well take a sugar pill as it has no effect whatsoever. It should be noted that buspirone does not treat panic attacks or obsessive compulsive behaviors. It is strictly used for generalized anxiety symptoms, such as worry, tension, feelings of apprehension, etc..

Side Effects

Buspirone is a nice medication. It has relatively low side effects. Being that it is a serotonin medication, we can expect nausea and stomach issues. Headache and dizziness are also reported along with some (very low) sedation. One of the benefits of buspirone is that there are no sexual side effects, which means that buspirone can be a good option for generalized anxiety over a traditional SSRI. Weight gain is also rare and not generally seen.

Mental Conditions Used For: Generalized Anxiety Disorder (GAD), some treatment-resistant depression

Anti-Histamines

Medication names: hydroxyzine (Vistaril, Atarax), diphenhydramine (Benadryl)

How does it work?

As the name suggests, antihistamines block histamine, which is a brain chemical that is responsible for arousal and alertness. When you get an allergic reaction, histamine runs wild, which is why your breathing can close off, you feel like you are panicking, and you have super anxiety. By blocking histamine, the body can calm down and reduce anxiety symptoms.

How long does it take to work, and what should I expect?

Anti-Histamines are taken "as needed" for high anxiety. These medications are taken by mouth and generally take 15-30 minutes to work. The effect should be quick, and you will know within an hour if the medication is working well for you.

Specific Differences

Hydroxyzine (Vistaril) - hydroxyzine is diphenhydramine on steroids. Typically regarded in some literature as 25x stronger than diphenhydramine, hydroxyzine is a good anti-anxiety medication. What is also nice about hydroxyzine is that it is not abusable and doesn't build any tolerance

Diphenhydramine (Benadryl) - diphenhydramine is often used for allergies, sleep, itching, and other uses. Generally, you'll see it used for sleep when people buy it from their local pharmacy. One issue with diphenhydramine to watch for is that it tends to lose its effectiveness over time.

Side Effects

Anti-Histamines are anti-cholinergic (there's that word again), which means it "dries" you up. This includes dry mouth, constipation, blurring vision, and sedation. Tremors have been seen but are more on the rare side. Adverse effects include convulsions, delirium, and slowing of breathing

Mental Conditions Used For: anxiety disorders, insomnia, agitation/violence, nausea

"Off label" Blood Pressure Medications

Medication names: propranolol (Inderal), clonidine (Catapres)

How does it work?

Propranolol is a high blood pressure medication that works by blocking beta receptors. Beta receptors, when turned on, are responsible for pumping norepinephrine and adrenaline in your body. This makes your blood pressure high, and heart rate increases. So, propranolol blocks these beta receptors, thus lowering norepinephrine and adrenaline. This helps with anxiety, especially panic attacks, because anxiety ramps up your body. This simply blocks the body from being raised to uncomfortable levels of anxiety.

Clonidine is seen in many "off label" usages. You will see clonidine in substance use detoxification and also in attention deficit hyperactivity disorder (ADHD). Clonidine is an alpha agonist, which means it turns on alpha receptors that help calm down the central nervous system. Calming the central nervous system helps with reducing blood pressure, but also reduces anxiety. Clonidine also reduces norepinephrine release in the prefrontal cortex (part of the brain that helps with focus, attention, decision making), which is why it can help with ADHD.

How long does it take to work, and what should I expect?

For both propranolol and clonidine, both should have more immediate effects (within 15-30 minutes). Propranolol is known to help reduce the physical manifestations of anxiety and panic attacks (pounding chest, sweating, difficulty breathing, numbness, etc.). Propranolol does not help the anxiety that is "in your head," meaning that it doesn't reduce the racing thoughts and worry thoughts. Nonetheless, for people with panic attacks, propranolol is a godsent as it can help relieve those uncomfortable panic symptoms. Clonidine is usually pretty immediate and generally works the same as propranolol. It's more sedating than propranolol, which may be better for more agitation than anxiety, as well as for sleep improvement.

Specific Differences

Propranolol (Inderal) - generally better for anxiety with physical symptoms. Help calm the physical body. It can be used in performance anxiety, such as giving speeches or concentration sports like archery. Propranolol is known to not be so sedating and keeps your brain with good ability to function, unlike other anti-anxiety medications that can sedate you.

Clonidine (Catepres) - seen more in use for agitated type anxiety. Its strong effects can be useful in substance withdrawal while also not lowering the heart rate as much as propranolol does.

Side Effects

For both propranolol and clonidine, dizziness and passing out can be common. This is due to it being a blood pressure medication. It can also cause dry mouth, constipation, and weakness. Headache and sexual side effects are also common. Propranolol can lower your heart rate to unsafe levels, especially at higher dosages. It should be noted that dosages for both propranolol and clonidine are generally much lower when used to treat anxiety compared to the dosages used to treat high blood pressure.

Mental Conditions Used For: panic disorder, anxiety disorders, post-traumatic stress disorder (PTSD), substance detoxification, agitation, and performance anxiety

Mood Stabilizers

Lithium

Medication names: Lithium (Eskalith, Lithobid)

How does it work?

Lithium is one of the oldest psychiatric medications in the world. It was actually stumbled on from trying to find a salt substitute. Lithium has been used for years to help people with bipolar disorder. It's interesting that for how long we have used it, we still don't understand exactly how lithium works in the brain. We know that it helps with regulating cells in the brain but other than that, we are not sure how it works. There is evidence of lithium reducing norepinephrine (stimulating brain chemical) and increasing serotonin (reduces impulsivity and gives a sense of well-being). There is also some evidence that suggest that lithium helps regulate glutamate, which is high in manic episodes of bipolar disorder. Lithium has neuroprotective benefits and helps the brain protect itself from stress and brain cell deterioration. There is new research looking at its role in traumatic brain injury and helping the brain preserve its functions.

How long does it take to work, and what should I expect?

Lithium is rather quick compared to other psychiatric medications. Generally, 1-3 weeks is the standard time frame we look at. Lithium is known for its side effects (not that everyone will experience them), so it's common for many people to drop lithium after a few days. Lithium is not necessarily known for its sedation, so you generally shouldn't feel sedated during the day. Expect to take a lithium level around five days after starting or changing the dosage of lithium. The lab needs to be drawn at least 12 hours after the last time taking lithium in order to get the correct level. Lithium is a lifelong medication, and it is known that if a person can stay on lithium adherently, the dosage or medication won't need to be changed for years, if ever.

Specific Differences

Lithium is a unique medication and of a class of its own. Being a natural salt, has specific differences compared to a lot of other psychiatric medications (some good, some bad). Lithium requires labs to see lithium levels. The lithium level is pretty narrow, which means that the level that actually starts to work in your body is relatively close to the level of toxicity, so monitoring labs is crucial. Lithium has this unique ability to be neuroprotective. The salt keeps brain cells from "popping" or dying. This can be very important in bipolar disorder as manic episodes typically have a lot of the brain chemical glutamate flowing. Glutamate is toxic to the brain and lithium can help prevent mania and also offset the damage. Lithium is one of two medications (the other being clozapine) that have substantial evidence of reducing suicidal thoughts and attempts. This can also be crucial for people with bipolar and treatment-resistant depression as it can help reduce these thoughts and impulses.

Side Effects

Wow! Lithium sounds so great! Why doesn't everybody get lithium? Side effects are the number one reason why lithium is underutilized or stopped by the person. Lithium is a salt, so urinating a lot and being thirsty are very common features. Nausea and diarrhea are the next most common side effect. A fine tremor can be a common occurrence with lithium. This can be alleviated with the medication propranolol. Another downside of lithium is the weight gain, which requires a real benefit to risk ratio analysis. Generally speaking, when you see lithium, it is usually because a lot of other psychiatric medications have been tried and have not worked. Most of these side effects dissipate with time as the body adjusts but can be very uncomfortable in the meantime.

Some of the more severe adverse effects of lithium can occur when toxicity is reached (above 1.4 mmol/L). This can include delirium, memory issues, and impaired coordination. Because lithium is a salt, high toxic levels can hurt the kidneys and cause heart rhythm issues. Long term lithium use (toxic or not) affects the thyroid, typically making it not put out enough thyroxine needed for your metabolism. Typically, long-time users of lithium will need to take supplemental synthetic thyroid medication to help keep the levels normal.

Despite the side effects, lithium is an excellent medication for bipolar disorder and treatment-resistant depression with suicidal tendencies. Closely monitoring the lithium level and adjusting dosages adequately can alleviate many of the side effects expressed above. I have seen many people's lives change for the better because of lithium, especially those with very severe bipolar disorder.

Mental Conditions Used For: bipolar disorder, treatment-resistant depression

Anti-Convulsant/Anti-Seizures/Mood Stabilizers

Medication names: valproic acid (valproate, divalproex, Depakote, Depakene), carbamazepine (Tegretol), oxcarbazepine (Trileptal), topiramate (Topamax), lamotrigine (Lamictal), gabapentin (Neurontin)

How does it work?

Anticonvulsant medications were all originally made to treat seizures. Seizures occur when the electrical system in your brain goes completely haywire, leading to detrimental shakes, freezes, and stops in thought. These medications work by not allowing the electricity to fire too much, thus preventing seizures. It does this by keeping in check the brain chemicals that ramp up the electrical system, mostly sodium, calcium, or glutamate, depending on the medication. Inadvertently, there are people who have seizure disorders, who also have bipolar disorder. When these people began taking anticonvulsants for their seizures, their mania and depression were also kept in check. By regulating the sodium channels, the brain is not able to rapid-fire, thus calming it. Anticonvulsants also show some action with serotonin and GABA (especially valproic acid), which helps with depression, anxiety, and impulse control.

How long does it take to work, and what should I expect?

Mood stabilizers can work comparatively quick compared to other psychiatric medications. In general, 2-3 weeks is the average trial time for mood stabilizers. By week 4, it should be apparent if the mood stabilizer will work or not. For acute mania episodes, you may see results within a few days. This makes mood stabilizers optimal for inpatient and rapid stabilization treatment. One should expect feeling less emotional volatility. If a person is manic, they may feel as if the "life of the party" is gone and may be irritable that they feel "flat" or "dull". In depression, reduction in symptoms is generally very welcomed.

Specific Differences

Valproic acid (Depakote) - valproic acid and lithium are by far the most used anticonvulsants in psychiatry. Valproic acid works very well with mania in bipolar disorder. It also is considered the best anticonvulsant for "rapid cycling" bipolar disorder (4 or more manic or depressed episodes a year). Valproic acid has a benefit of increasing GABA, which is a calming brain chemical. For this reason, it can be used for agitation, PTSD, and other impulse control issues. Valproic acid requires labs every few months to determine the level. The lab level for valproic acid is 50 - 100 mcg/ml. Valproic acid can be hard on the liver if the person is doing other intensive liver activities, such as drinking alcohol, so getting labs to test the liver is also important.

Carbamazepine (Tegretol) - this medication is a second line anticonvulsant used in bipolar disorder. Carbamazepine tends to be sedating like valproic acid, so it can help those who don't sleep well. One of the benefits of carbamazepine is that weight gain is usually not a feature, so if weight gain is seen in lithium or valproic acid, carbamazepine can be a good option to try. Carbamazepine is very well known for its interactions with other medications. For example, women on birth control need to know that if they take carbamazepine that their birth control may become ineffective. Always have your prescriber review your medications to ensure this doesn't happen. Carbamazepine can require labs depending on the provider and your uniqueness.

Oxcarbazepine (Trileptal) - the cousin of carbamazepine, oxcarbazepine works very similarly to carbamazepine and has, generally, the same results. What makes oxcarbazepine different is that it doesn't have some of the interaction issues that carbamazepine has. It also has less risk of some of the adverse effects of carbamazepine, such as low iron counts and other blood issues.

Topiramate (Topamax) - topiramate is a poor mood stabilizer. It's glory days (if I remember correctly) was the 1990s when it was first marketed. Topiramate is still used though to help with weight gain. This is an "off label" use, but it can help reduce appetite, and thus, weight gain. Topiramate's brand name is Topamax, and the long-time colloquial word was "dopamax," and that is because topiramate is very sedating. So, if you have insomnia, this is a great option. If you sleep too much, then this may be too sedating.

Lamotrigine (Lamictal) - lamotrigine is a common anticonvulsant used in bipolar disorder, as well as some depressions. Lamotrigine is not as effective for mania episodes, but it is very well known for help with bipolar depression or bipolar two disorder. This tends to be the bipolar type that is more depressed than manic, and when manic, tends to be hypomania, which is not as intense or impairing. Lamotrigine has to be titrated from the lowest dose to the optimal dose. This is because lamotrigine is known for a very rare, but very serious adverse effect called "Lamictal Rash." This rash forms on the skin when taking lamotrigine. If it happens, you call your prescriber immediately or as soon as possible and stop the medication (or follow your prescriber's instructions). This rash can lead to a serious and potentially deadly condition called Steven Johnson's Syndrome (SJS). Steven Johnson's Syndrome is a condition where an autoimmune crisis occurs, leading to the destruction of a layer in your skin that helps it hold to your body. This is completely avoidable if you watch for the rash and follow up with your provider. Generally, the rash will be frequently with flu-like symptoms, typically within 1-4 days of starting lamotrigine. Taper the medication slowly reduces the rate of this rash drastically. If the medication is stopped for 1 day or more, you have to start from the lowest dose again and titration up to the optimal dosage again. Even with this very rare adverse reaction, people tolerate lamotrigine very well most of the time. They generally tolerate it better than most other anticonvulsants, so don't let the "lamictal rash" scare you from an opportunity to feel better.

Gabapentin (Neurontin) - this medication is an anticonvulsant used in seizures, but also for nerve pain. Research shows gabapentin to be a weak mood stabilizer for bipolar. It is nonetheless used for bipolar disorder because it can help with anxiety and help with stabilizing the mood to some degree. Gabapentin is nice for people who have liver problems or maybe our problematic alcohol users. This is because gabapentin is easy on the liver, generally being all urinated out without much change.

Side Effects

Anticonvulsants have their share of side effects like most medications. Gastrointestinal issues are very common with all the anticonvulsants, which includes nausea and vomiting. Sedation is also very common with all the anticonvulsants. Weight gain can be problematic, with the exception of oxcarbazepine, lamotrigine, and topiramate. Dizziness may also occur.

Anticonvulsants and Pregnancy

Anticonvulsants are known to be harmful to fetuses when a woman is pregnant. It is vital that you inform your prescriber if you are trying to become pregnant. Generally, these medications will have to be stopped to maintain a healthy pregnancy, which can be scary because of the mental deterioration that may follow. It is still important to avoid any complications with your pregnancy that can be avoided in the first place.

Mental Conditions Used For: bipolar disorder, treatment-resistant depression, PTSD, anxiety disorders, traumatic brain injuries, and some personality disorders

Antipsychotics

Antipsychotics have an incredible stigma surrounding them. Indeed, the typical (first generation) antipsychotics have made the impression of making "zombies" out of everyone. And for those who have ever been inpatient or in the emergency department, you know that antipsychotics (typically the "typical" or first-generation) are used in injections to calm agitated patients. Because of this, people who very much need antipsychotics don't take them or even consider them. Antipsychotics are generally for psychosis, and as explained earlier in this book, psychosis can have a component where the person is not aware of their illness or has a deviation from reality. This makes taking antipsychotics (amongst other psychiatric medications) very difficult.

For how much antipsychotics get a bad rap, we can thank their invention for being the main driving force to shut down mental asylums and state hospitals (some may view this as a bad thing). Chlorpromazine, or Thorazine, was the first antipsychotic, first discovered in 1933 by accident when trying to find a new drug for allergies. Once chlorpromazine hit the market, it took over, and advocates began to lobby for the formation of community-based psychiatry rather than mental asylum type treatment.

From the side of the patient, it can be very understandable why taking an antipsychotic wouldn't be optimal. The side effects can be bad. It can rob you of the good feelings of mania in bipolar disorder, and it can feel like you aren't in control. Thoughts and perceptions are a human experience that can give tremendous meaning to our lives. That's what makes it different than taking lisinopril for your high blood pressure. Your blood pressure doesn't give you meaning, motivation, or understanding of the world, so taking medication for it isn't as powerful as one that can do the things that an antipsychotic can do, which is reduce delusions and hallucinations that can have meaning or powerful perceptions of their world. So much of the time, prescribers and people in the mental health community tend to forget this difference. For you or a loved one, always consider these common thoughts and stress that are faced when taking an antipsychotic. I, personally, almost always agree that a person who is psychotic will need to take an antipsychotic if they want to function well in the world, but that certainly doesn't mean it's easy for everyone to do so. Care and understanding are always foundational to medications and treatments like these.

Typical (First Generation) Antipsychotics

Medication names: haloperidol (Haldol), chlorpromazine (Thorazine), fluphenazine (Prolixin), perphenazine (Trilafon), trifluoperazine (Stelazine), thiothixene (Navane), thioridazine (Mellaril), molindone (Moban), mesoridazine (Serentil), loxapine (Loxitane). *there are others but are very rarely ever used anymore in modern psychiatry

How does it work?

Typical antipsychotics work by lowering the level of dopamine, a brain chemical that is theorized to be too high in the brain, which causes delusions and hallucinations. It does this by blocking the dopamine receptor D2. The D2 receptor needs to be blocked at least 65% or more. This means that there will be no reduction in hallucinations or delusions until this threshold is met. Typical antipsychotics work very well at blocking the D2 receptor but at the cost of lowering dopamine in other areas of the brain, causing the famous side effects that we hear of with these medications. The newer atypical antipsychotics have more selective parts in their mechanism but still, have side effects as well. Typical antipsychotics can lower dopamine in a part of the brain that deals with movement, which can cause tremors and movement issues that resemble Parkinson's disease. There is also a muscle freezing that can happen, where the muscles (typically starts on tongue or neck) become stiff. The lowering of dopamine in another area of the brain can also "flatten" a person's emotions, making them emotionless and with poor ability to socialize.

How long does it take to work, and what should I expect?

Typical antipsychotics generally work well and quick for hallucinations and delusions. Within one week, there should be some good effects. Side effects can show up within hours of taking an antipsychotic but can also take some time to develop if they are to. Typical antipsychotics work very well for "positive symptoms" of psychosis (hallucinations, delusions, disorganized speech). They do not work well and may even make worse "negative symptom" psychosis (emotionless, flat, poor social skills, isolation, poor motivation, poor attention, and poor speech abilities). Although we try the newer, generally fewer side effects, atypical antipsychotics first, we still use these typical antipsychotics for those who don't respond well to the newer atypical antipsychotics. There is no doubt that typical antipsychotics work very well for positive symptoms, generally over the newer atypical antipsychotics, so if the hallucinations or delusions are very impairing, that's when typical antipsychotics will be considered. Sometimes a small dosage is added to an atypical antipsychotic to help boost the dopamine lowering.

Specific Differences*

Covered typical antipsychotics below are the most commonly used typical antipsychotics used today. This isn't a comprehensive list of all typical antipsychotics

Haloperidol -the famous (or infamous) haloperidol, or Haldol. Well known in emergency rooms and psychiatric units across the world for emergency agitation. Haloperidol has been used for years for schizophrenia and other psychosis types and is the "go-to" for hallucinations and delusions that atypical antipsychotics aren't helping. One benefit of haloperidol is that it is not known for weight gain, which is almost universal in all other antipsychotics. Haloperidol is sedating and has a high incidence of extrapyramidal symptoms (EPS), which can include muscle freezing, tremors, internal restlessness, or little to no movements. This is usually offset by combining Benadryl or Cogentin (anticholinergic medications).

*Available as a long-acting injectable

Chlorpromazine -chlorpromazine was indeed the first antipsychotic ever made, and its contributions to the demise of the asylum systems in the U.S. are well known. Chlorpromazine is also known to be sedating and is still seen being used for emergency medications in emergency rooms and psychiatric units for out of control agitation. Interestingly enough, chlorpromazine also helps with nausea and vomiting. Chlorpromazine can have the side effects of extrapyramidal symptoms (EPS) but is much less known than haloperidol. It remains a very powerful medication for positive symptoms in psychosis (hallucinations and delusions).

Fluphenazine -fluphenazine is not used as much as its glory days but is still seen being used for some people. Generally, these people have been on fluphenazine for a long time and have been stabilized on it. The side effects are relatively the same as other typical antipsychotics

*Available in a long-acting injection

Loxapine -loxapine is a rather interesting typical antipsychotic, and that's because it may not even be a "typical" antipsychotic. There is some evidence that loxapine not only does what a typical antipsychotic does (blocks dopamine) but at lower dosages, may also increase serotonin. This is more like the newer atypical antipsychotics. Side effects are similar to most of the typical antipsychotics.

Perphenazine -like fluphenazine, perphenazine is not readily seen anymore unless the person has been on it for many years and is generally stabilized on it. It is a medication, like chlorpromazine, that is seen being used for nausea and vomiting.

Side Effects

Many of the typical antipsychotics are sedating, so side effects like sedation, dizziness, and potential weight gain are common. Many are "drying medications," meaning they can cause dry mouth, blurred vision, constipation, and difficulty for the bladder to release urine. Typical antipsychotics can raise a hormone in your body called prolactin. Prolactin (think lactating) is important in the formation of breast tissue and milk production. Some people who take typical antipsychotics may start growing breast tissue and even start to leak milk (men included). People who take typical antipsychotics at high doses or for a long time can get emotional deficit side effects. This includes blunted (or flat) expressions, little emotion, apathy, little motivation, and little pleasure in pleasurable activities. When we think about the "zombies" when people take psychiatric medications, this is what we are thinking of. This is on the rarer side, and even so, we don't use typical antipsychotics as primary treatment anymore, so this is becoming rarer and rarer as the research gets better.

There are some serious side effects that typical antipsychotics can cause that are very important to know. These can happen with atypical (newer) antipsychotics, but to a much lesser degree, making them the first line treatment for schizophrenia and psychosis.

Extrapyramidal Symptoms (EPS)

Extrapyramidal Symptoms (EPS) are a more common adverse effect of typical antipsychotics. They run on a spectrum from mild to very severe. EPS happens because the medication lowers the brain chemical dopamine too much in the areas of the brain that deal with movement. Generally, when EPS starts, it begins as a tightening of the neck or tongue. Sometimes a fine tremor will begin. Medications like Benadryl and Cogentin can help with these and generally can keep EPS from happening. If any EPS symptoms occur, go to your prescriber as soon as possible. It the freezing or difficulty swallowing occurs, then go to the emergency department or call 911. If the abnormal movements continue for a long time (years), people can develop a condition called Tardive Dyskinesia (TD), which is explained next.

Extrapyramidal Symptoms (EPS)	
Dystonia	Muscles tensing up or "freezing"
Parkinsonism	Rigid stance or "stiff" walking
Bradykinesia	Movements slow down
Tremor	Typically in arms, but also neck and trunk
Akathisia	Internal restlessness that is uncomfortable

Table 3.2 Extrapyramidal Symptoms (EPS)

Tardive Dyskinesia (TD)

Tardive Dyskinesia (TD) is a more permanent form of EPS. When antipsychotics are used for years (especially the typical, or older generation), TD is a possibility. In general, TD exhibits involuntary movements that look like jerking of the trunk of the body, or sometimes the mouth or neck. TD can present with "lip-smacking" or back and forth of the tongue in and out of the mouth. Good assessments by the prescriber include the Abnormal Involuntary Movement Scale (AIMS), which is used to assess if EPS is occurring and to treat the EPS to prevent TD. There are also two new (as of 2019) medications that are used to TD, which is a first in the mental health field. These medications are called valbenazine (Ingrezza) and deutetrabenazine (Austedo). Both these medications help keep more dopamine in the part of the brain that deals with movement.

Neuroleptic Malignant Syndrome (NMS)

Neuroleptic Malignant Syndrome (NMS) is another adverse effect that is important to know. Once again the typical (older) antipsychotics are more prone to NMS than newer atypical generation antipsychotics. NMS is caused, again, by too much lowering of the brain chemical dopamine in the brain. NMS is a medical emergency and needs to be treated in the emergency department, generally with a medication called dantrolene.

Neuroleptic Malignant Syndrome (NMS) Signs and Symptoms
Altered or delirious
Fever
Muscles become rigid (hard to move)
Sweating, high heart rate (above 100 beats per minute), and high blood pressure

Table 3.3 Neuroleptic Malignant Syndrome (NMS) Signs and Symptoms

Mental Conditions Used For: schizophrenia, bipolar disorder with psychosis, a major depressive disorder with psychosis, agitation, other psychotic disorders

Atypical (Second Generation) Antipsychotics

Medication names: asenapine (Saphris), quetiapine (Seroquel), olanzapine (Zyprexa), clozapine (Clozaril), risperidone (Risperdal), paliperidone (Invega), aripiprazole (Abilify), ziprasidone (Geodon), lurasidone (Latuda), cariprazine (Vraylar), brexpiprazole (Rexulti)

How does it work?

The invention of atypical antipsychotics was almost by accident. When clozapine (Clozaril) was created, it was aimed to be a typical antipsychotic. What ended up being created as the first atypical antipsychotic. Atypical antipsychotics still work by lowering the brain chemical dopamine in the brain, but with some added differences. Atypical antipsychotics help increase serotonin in parts of the brain that help reduce or even improve side effects typically seen in the older typical antipsychotics. This makes atypical antipsychotics having less prevalence of extrapyramidal symptoms (EPS).

Atypical antipsychotics can also help with schizophrenia that exhibits "negative symptoms," which is blunt looking, apathy, no pleasure, little to no emotion, and generally poor thinking skills. The increase in serotonin along with lowering of dopamine seems to help with negative symptoms, which older typical antipsychotics didn't even touch, or actually made worse. Newer antipsychotics even do better at decreasing side effects. Aripiprazole (Abilify) doesn't block dopamine like other typical and atypical antipsychotics, it more "regulates" how much dopamine is allowed in certain areas of the brain. Think of a dam that regulates the water flow. Traditionally, typical and atypical antipsychotics would be trying to put a stop to the flow, while newer antipsychotics like aripiprazole, would be allowing some water flow to stream out rather than trying to completely block it. This little allowance of dopamine can help reduce the rates of EPS and tardive dyskinesia. Because of the better side effect profile, we use atypical antipsychotics as first-line treatment in people with psychosis, like schizophrenia. Atypical antipsychotics do help reduce the more scarier side effects traditionally seen in typical antipsychotics, but atypical antipsychotics have their own set of side effects to watch out for. You'll read more about them below.

How long does it take to work, and what should I expect?

Atypical antipsychotics typically take less than a week to start helping psychosis (hallucinations and delusions). We should be mindful that delusions are typically harder to treat and, thus, may not be as apparent when looking at effectiveness. Even though atypical antipsychotics can start to work in less than a week, you want to see how it's working by weeks 4-6 as that is generally when the full effectiveness occurs. The same time frame can be said when using atypical antipsychotics for mania episodes seen in bipolar disorders. For depression, the results may take 2-4 weeks. For the person taking the medication, the effects can be subtle for psychotic symptoms. The person is much more likely to feel sedation if sedation is a major side effect of antipsychotics (quetiapine, asenapine, clozapine, olanzapine).

Psychosis in schizophrenia and schizoaffective disorder tend to be reduced when taking antipsychotics in general. It's actually on the rarer side that the psychosis (hallucinations and delusions) will go fully away. I always teach my patients that voices are like a radio that is too loud. Our job with medication is to turn down the volume to where the person can function in the world without too much distress. This is not to say that some people have complete remission of voices. This does happen, and thankfully so. It just tends to be on the rarer side, unfortunately.

Specific Differences

The "*-pines*" (**quetiaPINE, olanzaPINE, asenaPINE, clozaPINE**) - these atypical antipsychotics are very heavily used. They tend to be sedating, which can help people who are manic but also those who have sleep insomnia. These medications also tend to be associated with weight gain, a side effect that most people stop the medication because of. These medications also tend to be higher contributors to metabolic syndrome (increased blood sugar, increased weight, increased fat in the blood) than other atypical antipsychotics. They are nonetheless some of the best atypical antipsychotics we have for both mania episodes, treatment-resistant depression, and psychosis. Please read the note on clozapine (Clozaril) below to learn more about this atypical antipsychotic with special features

The "*-dones*" (**risperidone, lurasidone, paliperidone, ziprasidone**) - I like to consider these atypical antipsychotics as "middle ground," as they tend to be good, but not the strongest antipsychotics, and generally are in the middle of the side effect spectrum for antipsychotics. As such, they are good first-line treatments and for long term maintenance of psychosis and mania. Risperidone and paliperidone are almost identical to each other chemically wise, and both have a long-acting injectable option, which you can take every four weeks (Invega Sustenna). Lurasidone is a new and effective medication for bipolar depression. Lurasidone also has relatively low sedation and low weight gain, making it an optimal antipsychotic for weight-conscious people. Ziprasidone is also known for having little to no weight gain but is to be avoided if a person has heart conditions.

The "*-piprazoles*" (**aripiprazole, brexpiprazole**) - both these medications functions almost identically with the only difference being that brexpiprazole seems to have a longer time in the body (longer half-life). Both these medications are very good medications for bipolar and treatment-resistant depression. In fact, if a person with depression has not responded well to many antidepressants, sometimes we can throw a little aripiprazole and that enhances the antidepressant, both relieving anxiety and depression. They are both good at treating psychosis and people with bipolar disorder. One of the benefits of these medications is that they are known to not cause weight gain or have so much impact on the metabolic side effects seen in other atypical antipsychotics. The biggest and well-known side effect of aripiprazole is what is known as "akathisia" or internal restless energy that is very uncomfortable. Typically, going to the emergency room if it is very severe is needed, otherwise see your prescriber as soon as possible.

Cariprazine (Vraylar) -one of the newer atypical antipsychotics. Because it is so new, we don't have much long term data on the medication, but the research had shown some good results. Cariprazine's claim to fame is being a good dopamine regulator, too high (psychosis), it lowers it, too low (EPS), it raises it. This medication may be an advantage for people who exhibit negative symptoms seen in schizophrenia. It can theoretically help with bipolar disorders and bipolar depression.

Side Effects

What medication is without its side effects? (That includes natural substances too) Atypical antipsychotics are known to have a reduced chance of getting extrapyramidal symptoms (EPS), but nonetheless, people still can get EPS with the atypical antipsychotics. Atypical antipsychotics are known for their contribution to metabolic syndrome. Metabolic syndrome classifies as four different conditions - high blood pressure, high blood sugar, excess fat around the waist, and high cholesterol levels - and these can lead to detrimental health outcomes. Some of the atypical antipsychotics are more known for causing metabolic syndrome, most notably the "-pines" (olanzapine, clozapine, asenapine, quetiapine). Others are known to have a much smaller if no effect on causing metabolic syndrome (aripiprazole, brexpiprazole, lurasidone, ziprasidone). It is nonetheless something to monitor and keep a serious focus on. Lifestyle changes can dramatically help curb the effects of metabolic syndrome, including a diet high in plant type foods and daily exercise. Unfortunately, sometimes with schizophrenia or other psychotic disorders, there is a tendency to have little motivation to make such changes, so we must always weigh the risks and benefits of the side effects to the severity of the mental symptoms. Other more common side effects include dizziness, sedation (in select few), and some dry mouth, constipation, and increased thirst. Again, each antipsychotic has different side effects that are more common or less frequent than others, so it's always important to talk to your prescriber regarding the best decision.

Mental Conditions Used For: schizophrenia, bipolar disorder with psychosis, a major depressive disorder with psychosis, agitation, other psychotic disorders, mood-stabilizing in bipolar, treatment-resistant depression, treatment-resistant anxiety

A note on clozapine (Clozaril)

Clozapine, or Clozaril, is a well-known antipsychotic used for treatment-resistant schizophrenia or other psychotic disorders. Generally, when all other antipsychotics (both typical and atypical) have been tried, clozapine will be initiated and will generally work wonders for those who have had little to no success on any other medication. So why don't we just start with clozapine right off the bat? Clozapine is the last-line treatment for a reason. That reason is that clozapine can lower the white blood cells called neutrophils. Neutrophils are crucial for your immune system and are your first responders to any infection you get. Lowering neutrophils can be deadly because your body can't fight even the most basic of infections. When clozapine was first used, the mental health community was ecstatic! But soon, people were dying because of the lowering of neutrophils.

Years later (and lots of research), clozapine was allowed back on the market and now has one of the most stringent of requirements to use. What was found was that if you are slowing titrate (increase) the dosage over weeks, then the chances of lowering the neutrophils drops dramatically. Also, the U.S. government made a registry (Clozapine REMS), where a provider using clozapine has to register with the registry and put in every person that they put on clozapine. The person on clozapine then gives blood for lab work every week for the first six months, then every other week for the next six months, and then monthly after that for the duration of treatment. If the neutrophils drop below safe levels, clozapine is stopped immediately. Another safeguard is the pharmacy, which won't release the clozapine medication without updated lab work. Even though there are major side effects that can occur with clozapine, the monitoring and safety measures make it a relatively safe medication to use. Clozapine is also 1 of 2 medications (other being lithium) that is clinically known to reduce suicidal thoughts. Clozapine has really changed people's lives and shouldn't be discredited as an option, especially when all other antipsychotics are not working, and the person is suffering. The biggest factor is maintaining the appointments, lab work, and keep taking the medication daily.

Black Label Warning for elderly and dementia-related psychosis

Antipsychotics carry a black label, which is a risk label by the FDA in the U.S. The black label for antipsychotics is related to the risk of vascular (i.e., strokes, brain bleeds) in people who have psychosis (hallucinations, delusions) coming from their dementia. The risk is not actually as severe as the label comes across. Main studies point to a 1.6 times rate over placebo, which means that you are 1.6 times more likely to have this vascular issue than another person not taking antipsychotics. It should also be noted that there are people who have schizophrenia or other psychotic disorders that eventually get dementia (from genetic factors). These people can be treated with antipsychotics still and don't face the risk. The risk is involved with psychosis COMING from the dementia condition, not necessarily when there is dementia and differentiated psychotic disorder, like schizophrenia.

Novel and Other Treatment

Electroconvulsive Therapy (ECT)

ECT strikes fear into the hearts of many. Indeed, if there is a stigmatized treatment that people have seen scary movies of, it's with ECT. ECT involved placing electrical probes on the head and inducing micro seizures. We, of course, see in the movies a person going through ECT with the big mouth guard on and being shocked to the point of it being like they are on the electric chair. *One Flew Over the Cuckoo's Nest* exemplifies this perfectly when McMurphy goes through ECT as a punishment.

Why even "shock" the brain?

We first learned of shock therapy by accident through treatments relating to people with diabetics. Indeed, people with terrible depression who also had diabetes wouldn't care for their blood sugars and end up in low blood sugar seizures and convulsions. After being given emergency sugar into their blood, many would come out of the depression feeling much better. This led to research and the start of "shock therapy," which was used by injecting a depressed patient with insulin, dropping their blood sugar very low to the point of a seizure, then giving them sugar to bring them out of it. This is actually pretty horrifying to think of, but we have to remember that at the time, people were doing this because they honestly were trying to help people, not be sinister and purposely torture people. John Nash, the famous mathematician and key figure in the movie, *A Beautiful Mind*, went through insulin shock therapy. The therapy is actually portrayed in the movie. Eventually, researchers began looking at electrical shock as a way to stimulate the same response as insulin shock therapy, but without so much wear and tear on the body. Thus, ECT became a reality.

Since its beginnings, ECT has improved dramatically. The person is sedated and does not remember any of the procedure. The electrical voltage is tremendously lower than in the early days. The procedure is almost boring to watch because it seems that nothing is happening. Side effects are actually lower than many antidepressants; typically, some memory loss right after the procedure and an adverse effect is some longer-term memory loss (generally gaps of memories lost). These are still serious to consider, and that's part of the reason why ECT is a last resort treatment for chronically depressed or bipolar patients.

ECT generally is applicable for the person who has tried many treatments and therapies and has had no avail. Consent is always required unless the person is conserved or under guardianship. In California, to have ECT forced on someone, it takes four separate psychiatrists with no relation in their practice to assess and write reports on the necessary need for ECT. This is incredibly rare (I've only seen this tried once, and it didn't go through). ECT is a procedure, so you go into a operating suite and are put under general anesthesia. After the procedure, you are generally monitored by a nurse, mostly for sedation from the anesthesia. Sessions range from 5-10 sessions, then no treatment is needed. There are "tune-ups" that are sometimes done when the effects of the ECT wear off, but some may never need treatment again.

We have had ECT for decades now, and still, after all the research, we are not necessarily sure how it really works in the brain. Some theories point to brain protection measures, while others may have to do with blood flow or metabolism in the brain (maybe leading to more robust functions and brain chemicals?). The important aspect is that after decades of use, we know it is a very safe procedure and has little to no long term effects. We know that it's so safe that it is the recommended treatment for pregnant women with severe depression. The fetus remains healthy throughout the ECT. The success rate for ECT is about 50%, which sounds low, but to a person who has tried everything in the book to help their depression or mania, 50% is an amazing number! ECT is obviously not for everyone but maybe an underutilized treatment. It will become more or less used less frequently in the future as we move onto new and more efficient treatments.

Trans Magnetic Stimulation (TMS)

Trans Magnetic Stimulation (TMS) is a newer technology that we are slowing gathering data on for its effectiveness. TMS is similar to ECT but is definitely not ECT. TMS utilized powerful magnets to send magnetic waves into specific and focal areas of the brain that deal with depression. The magnetic ways are said to stimulate blood flow, metabolism, and electrical activity in the areas of the brain that help with uplifting depression. TMS has very little side effects, especially compared to medications. Generally, some people may have a slight, temporary headache after a TMS session. Very rare adverse effects include seizures and minor mania episodes. TMS success rates are still being researched, but 30% is a general marker for now. TMS is only approved for major depressive disorder at this time (2019), but research and implementation are being done for PTSD, negative symptoms in psychosis, and bipolar disorders.

Ketamine

Ketamine, long used as an anesthesia in emergency rooms and other areas in medicine that needed short term sedation, is now researched for depression. In many ways, the research on ketamine is showing that this may be one of the biggest breakthroughs in mental health treatment in years. Ketamine for depression has been released as esketamine (Spravato), which is a nasal spray that would be administered in the clinic by a licensed prescriber or nurse. Esketamine is only approved for depression and suicidal thoughts right now, but more and more research is looking into its use in other disorders (especially PTSD). Esketamine is known to increase dopamine, which helps with motivation and being able to experience pleasure. It also has been seen to increase blood flow, thus increasing function, in the prefrontal cortex, which helps with mood regulation and decision making. It also, and most importantly, works on NMDA receptors, which lowers glutamate. This is what causes dissociation when ketamine is abused, but at much lower dosages, this can help uplift depression. It will be interesting to see where the research leads us with ketamine as mainline mental health treatment. The future looks optimistic for this one.

9

THE PSYCHOTHERAPIES

"You are never too old to set another goal or to dream a new dream."
-**C.S. Lewis**

We Underestimate Therapy

Therapy can be profound in ways that no other mental health treatment can. Nothing can replace human interaction and connection. Therapy is more than just "talking about your childhood" or "think positive thoughts" (although these can be good strategies). Therapy has many modalities or types. Picking the right type for the mental condition is very important. Also, finding the right therapist that you can connect with and trust is very important. Psychotherapy in the United States healthcare system is always put on the back burners. Because of this, therapy is always seen as a "luxury" or it's not even offered as an option. This is tragic because we then miss out on a major piece of the pie to help ourselves or others with mental conditions. Understanding your past, facing your fears, building coping skills, decision making, different techniques to uplift yourself is only just a fraction of the benefits of therapy. We always hear, "a pill isn't going to fix it." There's some truth to this, especially for conditions like depression, anxiety, trauma, bipolar, and more. Medications help control the symptoms and can help increase functioning, which is very important. But therapy builds those tools, the understanding, and the ability to withstand future stressors, which can further protect your mental health. Therapy should always be considered for optimal care. The benefits really are so important that it would be unfortunate to miss out on the opportunity to gain from it.

Insurance Nightmare

One reason why psychotherapy is not usually an offered treatment option is because the health care system and insurance don't usually see psychotherapy as a primary option for mental health treatment. With quick, fast, and what they believe to be cheaper, medications and hospitals are the main treatments they like to fund. Because of this, finding a therapist can be difficult and costly. Even with the best insurances, challenges like prior authorizations, referrals, finding an insurance covered provider, providing the co-pay IF the insurance pays it can be more than a barrier, it can be an outright Great Wall of China. Insurances pose such an issue that many therapists simply won't take any insurance and do a "cash pay" only. This isn't because the therapist is cruel or money hungry, but the health insurance firms can make it a living nightmare to get the compensation needed for the therapy they provide. Imagine having to call and send notes back and forth for sometimes hours out of your day to maybe get denied reimbursement or get partial reimbursement. It's not only unfair to the therapist but undeniably a waste of their time for the training they received and DESIRE to help others with. Therapists are humans, too, and they do need to earn a living that is as stable as possible just like the rest of us. Unfortunately, therapists are also grossly underpaid for the benefits they provide, especially if doing their treatment through health insurance. Doing "cash pay" is a means to simplify the part of the job that we (all mental health providers) hate doing which is asking for compensation for our services. It also lessens their times on the phones or on the computer tailoring all their notes or fighting with the health insurance to get properly reimbursed. I know, I know, this isn't your problem, and I'm not writing this to make us all feel terrible for therapists. This merely encapsulates the barriers that hold people back from receiving the services they need to help their mental health.

Costs for "out of pocket" or "cash pay" vary. Generally, $65 - $300 a session is a good estimate to the range for therapy without insurance. Some initiatives have been started to help make therapy more affordable to people. These initiatives, like Open Path Collective (www.openpathcollective.org) offer therapy for an initial $49 sign-up fee and $30 - $60 per session. These sessions are generally being performed by unlicensed therapists getting their hours for licensure, but rest assured, they are qualified, being supervised, and (honestly) can be really good because they have the newest and greatest research from their recent schooling.

Please note that some therapists also offer a "sliding scale." This allows the therapist to adjust their session rate to a rate that is more affordable to you. This is always up to the therapist to do a sliding scale and is not mandatory for them to do so, but always inquire and see what they offer.

What does the best evidence say?

There has been a tremendous amount of research regarding the separate use of psychotherapy and medications, and then psychotherapy with medications together. The general consensus from all this research suggests that using both medication and psychotherapy have a synergistic effect compared to either one alone. What does this mean? There is a double value you get with coupling psychotherapy and medications, which enhance each other more than if only one was done alone. There are times that medications help bring someone into the "therapeutic window," which is a state where they are mentally healthy enough to engage and prosper in therapy. If you have daily panic attacks or in bed all day with terrible motivation, then you may not engage in therapy or even benefit from it if it were given to you in your house. The other side is that therapy can be beneficial but correspond with medication allowing for emotions to not run so wild, which then allows the therapy skills to be more effective as the severity is not as strong. Either way, choosing to do psychotherapy, medications or both is a personal choice and one that you have to remain comfortable engaging with. Evidence also shows that some mental conditions also respond better to therapy (notably the anxieties and depressions) than say other mental conditions (schizophrenia, bipolar) because of the brain-based nature of these disorders. Always consult with a mental health professional to be assessed and geared towards the best possible treatment for you.

The Therapies

Cognitive Behavioural Therapy (CBT)

Introduction

We start with cognitive behavioral therapy (CBT) for a good reason. It is one of the most, if not the most, used psychotherapies used in the world. Its format and structure are very adaptable, leading it to be used for a whole array of mental issues, from anxiety, depression, trauma, insomnia, and even eating. CBT started with the marriage of cognitive theory and behavioral theory. Aaron Beck is considered the father of CBT. CBT is very well researched and its ability to help create real change is nothing short of miraculous for most people. The goal of CBT is to focus on your thoughts and to challenge the validity of them. CBT works on the framework that our thoughts can be distorted with reality, which can lead to strong emotional distress and behaviors that are not conducive to our wellbeing.

How Does It Work?

Cognitive Behavioural Therapy (CBT) works on the CBT triangle - Thoughts - Emotions - Behaviours (see figure 4.1). Thoughts can be distorted by the nature of our human mind. These "cognitive distortions" then lead to emotions that are matched with the distortion, but not with reality, this leads to behaviors that are mismatched or not adaptive to the reality of your stressor or issue.

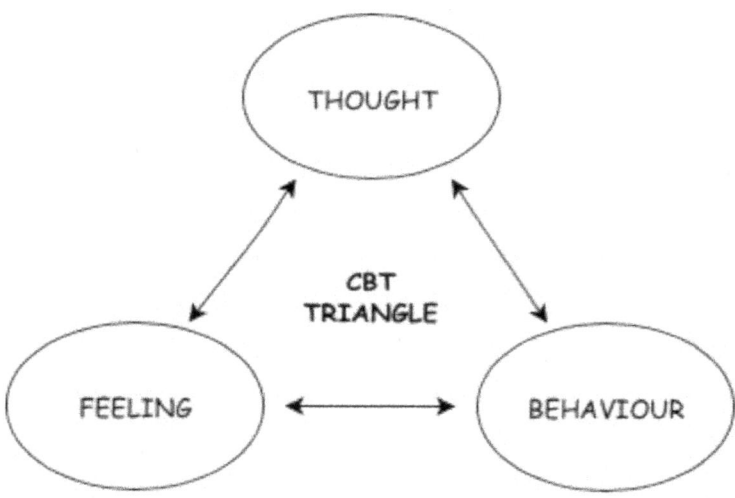

Figure 4.1 The CBT Triangle

An example could be you feel very anxious about an exam. Your thought is, "if I fail this exam, then I'm stupid." Now a statement like that is very concrete, and it's also "black and white" (distortion) thinking or "all or nothing" (either pass or be stupid, no other ways to think about it). Those thoughts lead to more anxious emotions and more stress, which overwhelms you. This can lead to the behaviors of procrastination or avoidance to not face the emotionally loaded studying for the exam. This, then, can lead to under preparation and actually not doing well on the exam. This, unfortunately, will reinforce the original thought that "you are failure," which then makes you anxious for the next exam and so on. Now say, you challenge that original thought: "If I were to fail the exam, would I be stupid?"

Some answers may be "well not really because I've made it this far and done a decent job" or "what does it even mean to be stupid?" A challenge I give people is, "if a friend you deeply care for said that if they fail the exam, then they would be stupid," and they were feeling distressed over it, would you completely agree with them on that statement? You would most likely challenge that thought, say, "of course you wouldn't be 'stupid,' exams are a matter of studying and learning the material." You may also say, "you are not stupid, you have done so many things that are not 'stupid.'" Why do we hold that double standard for ourselves? Why do we not allow ourselves to be kind and loving to our stressors as we would for a friend or family member we love? If you really can't find an answer to that, then maybe we need to focus on self-esteem, self-compassion, and confidence.

Now, you've challenged that thought of "If I fail the exam, then I am stupid." You identified the "black and white" distortion and also the "all or nothing" distortion. You then allow the thought of "If I fail the exam, that wouldn't be optimal, but I wouldn't be stupid." This can disarm the strength of the anxiety from the exam. Suddenly, the exam seems more manageable because it isn't loaded with these harsh and powerful statements. This lowers your anxiety (emotion), which then makes the behavior of studying more practical and feasible. You then study for the exam and get a decent to good grade on it. This is just one example of hundreds, if not thousands of examples that CBT can help with. CBT can deal with the simple test anxiety to the most complex of feelings and emotions from deep traumas and substance use.

List of Cognitive Distortions
All or Nothing - "I can only get 100% on this test or else I fail" **Mind Reading** - "They think I'm a failure" **Emotional Reasoning** - "I feel stupid, so that means I am stupid" **Personalization** - "that comment she said must have been about me" **Labeling** - "the exam didn't turn out well; I always fail at anything I try to do" **Catastrophizing** - "if I go to work, I'm definitely going to be yelled at" **"Should" Statements** - "I SHOULD have known better" **Overgeneralization** - "everything goes wrong for me" **Control Fallacy** - "if I'm not in complete control all the time, I will go out of control" **Comparing** - "I'm not as good as the other people here" **Disqualifying the Positive** - "she said I looked pretty, she obviously is just being nice and doesn't mean it" **Perfectionism** - "I have to do this perfectly or else it's a complete failure" **Filtering** - "I need to focus on all the bad and not focus on the good because the good doesn't matter" **Unrealistic Expectations** - "I must be the best at all times"

Table 4.1 Cognitive Distortions in CBT

What Should I Expect?

Cognitive Behavioural Therapy (CBT) typically consists of 8-15 sessions depending on the given issues being faced. Typically, the first session will be history taking and narrowing down the most prominent symptoms. The next sessions will focus on teaching CBT methods. Everyone who has done CBT knows that there is homework. Between sessions, you'll fill out mood logs, downward arrow technique sheets, and many more. These are to help reinforce the CBT skills learned. CBT is a "practice makes perfect" therapy, so practicing the skills is an important function of the therapy's success. CBT can always be continued after the initial sessions. Many people have more than "1" fear or "inadequacy," so frequent visits can help tackle those distortions.

Psychodynamic Therapy

Introduction

Psychodynamic theory picked up its roots from Sigmund Freud's psychoanalysis in the 19th century. The psychodynamic theory focuses on past events, along with conflicts in the "psyche" of the brain. Typically, these focus on the ID, Ego, and Superego. The ID refers to the part of the psyche that is primal, lustful, immediate gratification, and violent. The Ego if you play between the ID and superego. Its goal is to balance the two extreme worlds of the ID and superego. The superego is your societal and cultural standards that are pressured by the self to maintain. These conflicts and interaction between these three parts of the psyche is unconscious according to psychodynamic theory, and thus lead to the symptoms we see in depression, anxiety, and other mental health issues. The goal of psychodynamic therapy is to recognize, label, and remedy the unconscious conflicts. It does this through ranges of exploring past events (especially in childhood), to free association (sporadic random words and the first thought that comes to mind) and identifying transference and defense mechanisms. Transference is when you meet someone for the first time, and you (maybe even not acutely aware) judge or have a certain perception of the person based on past people or events.

An example could be my sister having a borderline personality disorder. Having grown up with a sister with a borderline personality disorder, I have formulated some thoughts and ideas about borderline personality disorder. So, in the future, I meet a person who does some behaviors that resemble borderline personality disorder (or maybe they tell me they have a borderline personality disorder), and my mind reacts with a perception of "how that person is and will be." Learning about transference is important for anybody as it can help lead to how you view others and what little triggers you have towards certain ideas or events. Psychodynamic therapy thus uses methods to help bring awareness to these unconscious thoughts to give you the power to understand and not fight them.

How Does It Work?

Psychodynamic therapy is generally a long term therapy. Most of the time, the person will have psychodynamic therapy for a least one year, and most of the time, longer. Part of this is due to how psychodynamic therapy works. It takes tremendous amounts of time to examine the past and the thoughts of the unconscious. Although there is some evidence that psychodynamic therapy for less than a year is moderately beneficial. This is actually more time-efficient than the old psychoanalysis, which took years and years to get anywhere (insurances don't like that kind of treatment). Typically, today, you will see and experience psychodynamic therapy as a part of other psychotherapy methods used (CBT, ACT, etc.). This blended method allows for the person to benefit from psychodynamic therapy while harnessing new tools to help deal with the now.

What Should I Expect?

Psychodynamic therapy uses a multitude of techniques to bring out the unconscious and explore the psyche conflicts. Analysis and thoughts about your dreams or fantasies may be used. You may also do "free association," where you just allow any thoughts and words to come out freely without any interruption from the therapist. The idea is that your thoughts and the words you say are connected to the deeper unconscious issues you may be having. Being able to engage these unconscious thoughts allows you to release repressed emotions and feelings that drive your everyday behaviors that may (or not) be hindering your mental health. I know of many people who didn't necessarily have a "mental illness" but did psychodynamic (or psychoanalysis) to simply learn more about themselves and their drives in life. For many, gaining the clarity of how your brain operates with thoughts and emotions can give you the ability to help control them in the future, which can be uplifting.

Dialectical Behavioral Therapy (DBT)

Introduction

Dialectical Behavioral Therapy (DBT) was created by Marsha Linehan, a top researcher at the University of Washington and a fellow sufferer of borderline personality disorder. She wanted to create a therapy that would help those who had chronic suicidal thoughts, along with mood disturbances. DBT is the combination of distress tolerance skill building, mindfulness, emotional regulation, and interpersonal effectiveness. These four main topics are important in the treatment of borderline personality disorder, for which DBT is one of the only therapies that shows effectiveness in treating. DBT has also extended to help other mood disorders, just as trauma, PTSD, depression, anxiety, substance use, and bipolar disorder. DBT's roots are in cognitive behavioral therapy (CBT), so you generally will see many CBT skills employed with DBT. DBT just has added features that make it more comprehensive for those with emotional and mood dysregulation.

How Does It Work?

Dialectical Behavioral Therapy (DBT) has both individual sessions and skills building groups. The individual sessions are geared towards the personal needs of the person. The therapist will work to provide encouragement, clarity, motivation, and tailor specific obstacles that someone may be facing. The skills-building groups are focused on learning DBT skills and doing homework during the week. The group also provides companionship, a sense of belonging, and a chance to learn from others who struggle with the same issues. DBT consists of these two different modules so that the person can benefit from all the researched back interventions in traditional therapy. The skills range between the four main topics expressed above. These can range from mindfulness training and being present, to interpersonal relationship communication skills with boundary learning, to learning how to change unwanted thoughts and behaviors and more.

What Should I Expect?

A person should expect to be doing sessions weekly for at least six months. DBT is a dedication and investment, but the rewards are tremendous. Each skill learned in DBT is adaptable to many life situations and builds resilience and better relationships. Expect weekly homework, including Diary Cards and mood logs. These are important for incorporating the newly learned skills into practice with specific real-world situations and stressors. Groups can be very uplifting, but feeling nervous is completely normal. It should be noted that people in DBT can drop out due to unforeseen stressors or perceived inability to complete the DBT sessions. Expect the concepts and skills to feel "awkward" at first. These are new ways of thinking about yourself and the world, a deviation from what you have normally been doing. Change is always a challenge, but remember that you are investing in yourself and that is incredibly important for your wellbeing.

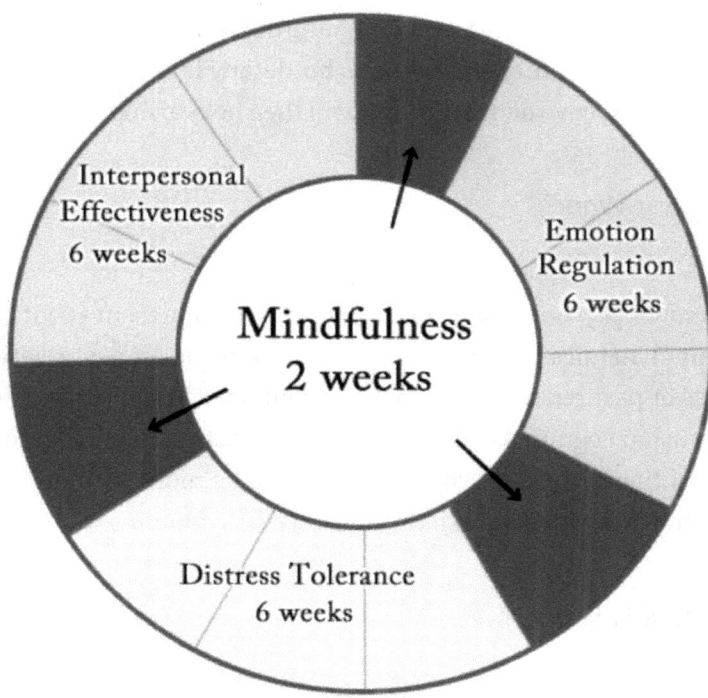

Figure 4.2: Breakdown of DBT Topics and Schedule

Interpersonal Psychotherapy

Introduction

Interpersonal psychotherapy is an adaptive therapy that focuses on improving social relationships, relational distress, and help with grief involved in major life transitions or events (divorce, death of loved one, bankruptcy). The goal is for a new understanding of ways to better foster relationships with close ones and how to resolve ongoing distress from major life events. The main theory of interpersonal psychotherapy is that you can improve upon your social environment, which will then help to improve your mood.

How Does It Work?

Interpersonal psychotherapy generally focuses on present events and relationship dynamics. There is typically not a focus on past relationship dynamics or past relationships that had conflict. The approach is focused on skills using cognitive and behavioral approaches, much like cognitive behavioral therapy (CBT). The focus tends to be more on improving the relationship than working on individual mental symptoms.

What Should I Expect?

Generally, interpersonal psychotherapy is a time-limited therapy. 10 to 15 weeks is a common time frame for interpersonal psychotherapy. Sessions typically consist of identifying problem areas and working on skills to improve upon these areas. Like CBT, there is generally homework that is to be done during the week. This is to reinforce the skills learned and gives a wonderful chance to use those newly learned skills in the individual's real-world stressors. Interpersonal psychotherapy tends to be either individual sessions or group sessions, depending on the provider.

Acceptance and Commitment Therapy (ACT)

Introduction

Acceptance and Commitment Therapy (ACT) is a well-versed psychotherapy used by many clinicians today. ACT started in the early 1980s and has since shown efficacy for stress, anxiety, depression, and other mental conditions. Its origins are based on mindfulness and cognitive acceptance of strong emotions we face. Originally, ACT was named *cognitive distancing* by its founder, Dr. Steven C. Hayes. The idea was that you wouldn't grapple with strong emotions head-on, but rather *distance* yourself from the feelings and accept them for what they are. Generally, grappling with strong emotions is an attempt to try and get rid of them, which usually ends in frustration and impulsive behaviors that are not in line with our goals and values.

How Does It Work?

ACT's main focus is on accepting your current state and then moving towards a behavior or action that is in line with your values and goals. According to the ACT theory, strong emotions can elicit strong reactions to them, which can lead to decisions and actions we regret later. These decisions and actions may make the feelings worse, or worsen the situation causing the strong emotions.

A great way to remember the ACT process is by the following:
    Accept your reactions and be mindful (present) with them
    Choose a valued direction
    Take the appropriate action

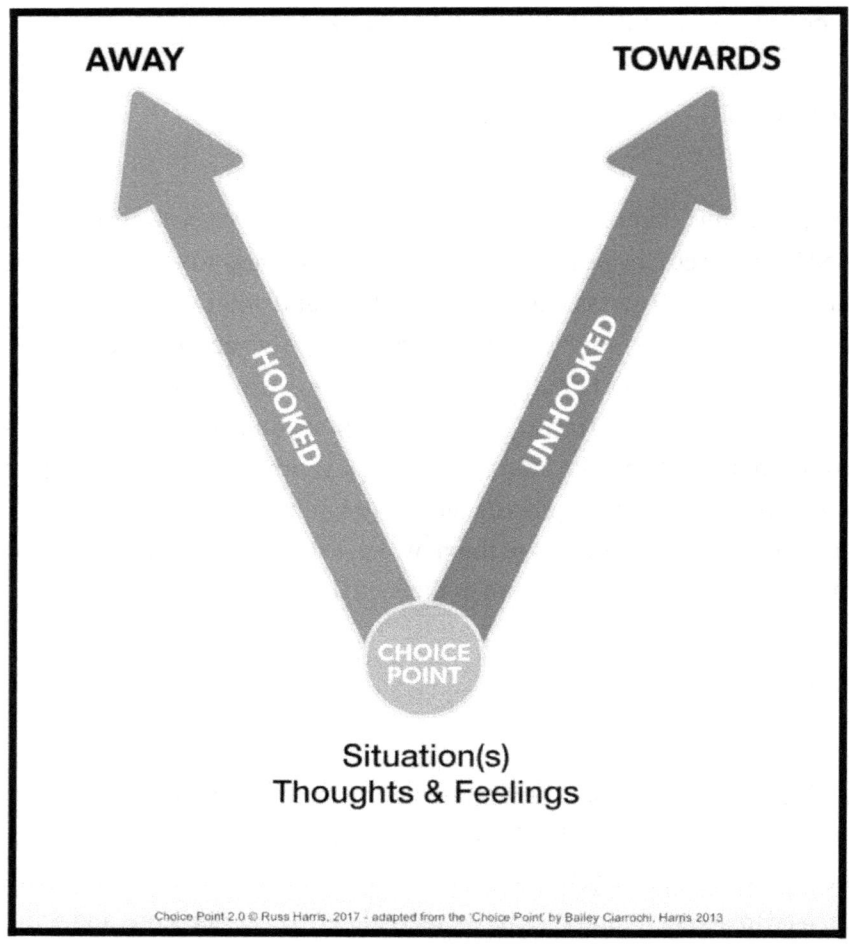

Figure 4.3 ACT Therapy works on your decision making by working towards your values

The goal is to *defuse* the strong emotions and to make more informed choices based on reality and your values. The ACT consists of 6 processes, or steps, that are the core of the practice. These include:

1. Defusion
2. Acceptance

3. Awareness
4. Transcending
5. Values
6. Committed Action

It's important to note that the values that are aimed for in ACT are the values that you have created for yourself. This makes the decision making stronger and gives you more of a brain reward for making decisions that align with your values.

What Should I Expect?

Like most therapies, the first session is generally an intake. This can be exploring what brought you to therapy and the key target symptoms that you want to focus on. For some, it may be depression, while for some, it is anxiety, or OCD. The ACT techniques are new, so the therapist will then help guide you to recognize your own emotions and learn how to listen to your own thoughts. This then leads to being able to identify difficult and debilitating emotions. Once one starts to recognize these emotions, they then can be guided with the ACT process above: defusion, acceptance, awareness, transcending, values, and committed action. The ultimate goal is to build more mental flexibility, or resilience to stress and strong emotions. This can then lead to increased confidence and self-esteem. ACT can be performed individually, or in group settings with good efficacy.

Cognitive Processing Therapy (CPT)

Introduction

Cognitive Processing Therapy (CPT) is a trauma therapy that is widely used for veterans with post-traumatic stress disorder (PTSD). The Veteran's Administration (VA), thus, researches CPT and its effectiveness with trauma and PTSD. We have some of the best evidence for CPT and its ability to help people with traumatic experiences. CPT falls in line with other trauma therapies that involve facing and engaging with the traumatic memories. In general, traumatic memories are naturally avoided because they cause such distressing thoughts, emotions, and behaviors. CPT allows the person to tell the story and build coping skills to handle the emotional distress that can follow. As you can imagine, CPT has a low engagement rate, meaning that many people either don't want to do it or drop out during the sessions. This is because CPT is uncomfortable, anxiety-provoking, and almost "unnatural" to what your body wants to do with the traumatic memories (which is to avoid them). It is NOT because of a lack of backbone, poor motivation, or denial. These are really painful memories that wreak havoc and rob the person of any normalcy in daily life.

How Does It Work?

CPT involves learning about a person's trauma symptoms. This can array from high anxiety, self-blame, guilt, easily startled, isolation, and more. Being educated on these symptoms gives clarity on why these emotions happen. The next phase works on writing down the more severe traumatic memories. Here, your brain begins to try to avoid the subject and gives you those strong emotions because it believes it may be occurring again. Over time, as the story is read, periodic stopping of the reading is done to identify the strong emotions and thoughts behind them. Through enough re-telling of the story, the brain "normalizes" the story (not that the trauma experience was normal!), but it makes the brain not as reactive to those memories. Retelling the story in a safe space with learning coping skills teaches your brain that these traumatic events had a beginning and an end and that they are not still occurring. This can release the brain's attempts to react and feel as if the trauma will happen again.

What Should I Expect?

The first session(s) are generally related to education about trauma symptoms. You learn about your specific trauma symptoms and why they generally occur. Next, expect to identify and write down your most traumatic memory. This is very challenging for anybody and generally takes a lot of time to accomplish (if accomplished at all). The subsequent sessions are the retelling of the story, while the therapist stops you periodically to help identify feelings and emotions, along with thought disturbances. Through this process, you will learn techniques for coping and get to practice them when not in therapy. Conclusively, there is education regarding the further development of adaptive skills to future stressors. CPT generally is 12 sessions, although it can be extended or done again for other traumatic memories.

Prolonged Exposure Therapy

Introduction

Prolonged Exposure Therapy (PET) is along the same lines as cognitive processing therapy (CPT), in that it's a type of exposure therapy. As we know, with trauma and PTSD, some triggers or sights can incite fear, anger, and outright feelings of being out of control. PET seeks to slowly expose you to these triggers in order to desensitize the trigger. As you can imagine, PET can be very uncomfortable and downright scary for some. To face the fears that you have been struggling with is incredibly brave and courageous.

How Does It Work?

PET works by exposing the person to a trigger. For example, a combat veteran is triggered when riding or seeing a Humvee military vehicle because it is what he was riding in when he and his fellow soldiers hit a roadside bomb. PET would allow the combat veteran to do exposure to elements that resemble the Humvee. This may be diesel smell or even virtual reality computers that have him ride in a Humvee. During this exposure, a therapist works through the strong feelings and emotions to help build awareness and coping skills to the event. This is typically done using cognitive behavioral techniques to help see the thought - emotion - behavior connection. Over time, the brain begins to learn that this traumatic event is over, and the brain (and body) can start to relax. PET is generally seen with military veterans and typically in Veteran Administration (VA) facilities, although there are places that specialize in these types of exposure therapies.

What Should I Expect?

Generally, PET has 15 sessions in total. There are two types of PET techniques, one being imagine-based and the other being *in-vivo* based. Imagine-based is as it sounds. It involves telling and re-telling of the story, which is the main part of the therapy. Periodically, when the person gets too overwhelmed, cognitive behavioral techniques are used to explore this. In Vivo is the use of actual items or virtual reality technologies to recreate elements similar to the traumatic experience. As you can imagine, it is very tough to do either one of these types of PET. Around 10-30% of people who start PET won't finish the full 15 sessions. Evidence does show that PET is very effective. Around 80% of people who complete PET sessions have a positive benefit and some relief from their trauma symptoms.

Eye-Movement-Desensitization and Reprocessing (EMDR)

Introduction

EMDR began its roots in the 1980s and has since grown into one of the most effective psychotherapies for trauma and PTSD. It has skyrocketed to be one of the premier trauma therapies, even being used with veterans with PTSD in the VA. Some data shows that EMDR therapy for a single trauma event (car accident, hurricane, etc.) can have 77 - 100% reductions in symptoms by six sessions. Complex trauma, or multiple traumatic events, are more challenging to remedy, but EMDR still provides excellent efficacy for complex trauma symptoms. Another benefit of EMDR is that it generally has fewer dropout rates compared to other trauma therapies. As discussed before, trauma therapies are very challenging. Generally, you are to revisit the traumatic events head-on and desensitize to them. EMDR is met with some controversy in the trauma therapy world, and it is mostly unfounded. EMDR is not very well understood on how it works, and when we don't know how something works, we don't like that because we like to know how things work to support them. Even with not understanding exactly how EMDR helps trauma symptoms, it is a very effective and safe therapy for trauma and PTSD, and there is no doubt that as we have plenty of research to expound that.

How Does It Work?

We are not sure how EMDR works. We do have ideas, though. Trauma and PTSD is usually a disconnect between your emotional center (limbic) and your memory center. Because a trauma event fragments and chops up memories of the trauma, the emotional center tends to not understand the event and is constantly pressed "on" and working to fight the next attack. This disconnection can wreak havoc on the person, whose brain doesn't know that the trauma has ended and can focus on other matters. It is suggested that EMDR, with its physical movement of the eyes while holding mental images or stories of the trauma, helps to connect these two systems. Once the memories are consolidated, the brain may learn that the trauma is not occurring anymore; it has a beginning and an end. When it learns that, the brain's emotional center can begin to calm and gain control. Research does show that the prefrontal cortex (impulse control/decision making) is highly activated during EMDR, while the fear center (amygdala/limbic) is inhibited. This is precisely what you want to help calm the fires of trauma symptoms.

What Should I Expect?

EMDR has 8 phases, each building on each other. Phase 1 will contain history gathering and learning, which traumatic experiences are the most distressing. This is where you and the therapist determine which trauma memory or story to focus on first. Phase 2 involves the preparation for battle; that is, you will learn coping and emotional techniques to help with very difficult emotions. These are to help with the distress that can occur during the next phases. Phase 3 - 6 are the actual telling or holding mental images of the traumatic event. While performing these actions, the therapist periodically will have you look at their finger and follow it with your eyes, side to side. This also may be done with bilateral pulsing controllers that pulse from one to the other and back. Phase 7 works on daily logs that focus on weekly distressing moments, the triggers, and which coping skills help the most. This is to help learn and filter through the coping skills to learn to work for any particular triggers or distressing emotions. The last, phase 8, is the concluding session that recaps all the comprehensive treatment performed along with tips on how to seek help if any trauma symptoms were to arrive again. EMDR can be useful in other conditions other than trauma, as well. Some evidence shows that depression, anxiety, substance use, and more can benefit from EMDR therapy. The future's looking good for such a powerful therapy.

Family and Couples Therapy

Introduction

We are social creatures; the kind that enjoys being with others and forming bonds. These relationships help out mental health more than we can ever imagine. But, with relationships comes potential strain, stress, and outright ugliness. When these events happen, family and couples' therapy can provide the skills needed to foster the relationship more. Family and couples therapy is one of the more known therapies available. One of the major challenges of family and couples' therapy is simply being able to orchestrate everyone that needs to be there to actually be there and get engaged. As you can imagine, if you are considering family and couples therapy, it may be because working together is a struggle already, so getting "buy-in" from other member(s) along with participation may be a challenge right from the start.

How Does It Work?

Family and couples therapy is a very broad concept in and can have many faces to it. Family and couples in the mental health system actually constitute their own field of study because the information, therapies, and dynamics are so vast. In its most basic form, family and couples therapy focuses on the dynamics, or relationship, between the persons. Some focus may include looking at communication styles. Maybe one person is very good at expressing their feelings while another is not, leading to feelings of disconnect or not feeling valued. It could be that the dialogue between people is full of insults or degrading comments that are superficial but lead to deep hurt or feelings of inadequacy in the relationship. Being able to have a trained eye observe these conversations can help to pinpoint the underlying beliefs and then work with changing those beliefs to make a more productive and fruitful relationship. When children are involved, there are more dynamics and there is a need to understand where everyone is developmentally in their understanding of relationships and family. Sometimes child behaviors maybe not what they seem due to the family dynamics. For example, a kid may break a plate, hit their sibling, throw a tantrum, which would then lead to a parent (or both) attending to the child and giving some sort of punishment or consequence. Now is this because the child desires attention from a parent because they feel neglected and they don't care if it's positive or negative attention? Maybe the child acts out in this way so that they don't have to see both parents fighting each other, even at the expense of their wellbeing. Is it bullying at school? Something else we can't even put our finger on? The array of reasons can seem daunting even to those who are thoroughly trained to help with these types of issues. Bowen's Family Systems theory is one of the more prominent backgrounds in family and couples therapy. Bowen's Eight Concepts of Family Systems (Figure 4.3) is a framework that family and couples therapy used for the general understanding of how relationships work, along with how they don't work.

What Should I Expect?

Venturing into a new environment to talk about your most heated and sensitive topics can be daunting and frightening. Merely making the first step into the office is a brave move and half the battle. Generally, the first session consists of getting to know the members, along with setting "ground rules." These "ground rules" tend to be how communication is to occur during the sessions. This is to start the journey to constructive communication and to reduce any hostility. The "ground rules" tend to focus on the reduction of "name-calling," judgments, time outs, patience, listening, and more. Sometimes the therapist may want to talk to each person separately at certain points. This is not to "gossip" or to "talk behind you back," but simply to allow the other person to open up honestly in a more neutral environment.

Bowen's Eight Concepts of Family Systems	
Triangles	A three person relationship (ex: two parents and child). Can create tension due to "odd man out" or "outsider" feelings
Differentiation of Self	Creating a sense of self is important in understanding your role in any family. A poor sense of self may lead one to be heavily reliant on others, or heavily influenced by what others think of them
Nuclear Family Emotional Process	Tension arising from long term tension between one or more members. This could be related to marital conflict, spouse dysfunction, child impairment, or emotional distancing
Family Projection Process	Projection in families comes when the parent projects their emotional issues to their offspring. This can cause extra pressure and anxiety in a child who is trying to bear adult emotional issues
Multigenerational Transmission Process	Generations operate to transmit emotional regulation and cultural norms in relationships. For couples, it's important for their to be a "matching" level of sense of self, meaning their views of independence from others
Emotional Cutoff	When problems or tensions are not resolved over time, a family may emotionally cut off a member or members. This is an attempt to reduce the tension
Sibling Position	Theory that position, or sibling order, has effects on the roles they will take. For example, an older sibling taking on more leadership roles, while the youngest may become demanding for being in charge or becoming dependent
Societal Emotional Process	This describes how society is governed by emotional processes that are familiar to a family. It also focuses on how society interacts with families and the conclusions they make about families ("their parents must be terrible because their kid is a bully")

Table 4.2 Bowen's 8 Concepts of Family Systems

Being as honest and transparent is the key to effective and fruitful therapy. In families, children may be talked to individually or as a group sometimes. This may lead to separating the parents to talk to them individually. One thing I frequently see with any couples or family therapy is generally one person has the main motivation to start the therapy. Generally, this is the person who feels that the *other* person is the one who needs the therapy more and they see themselves as more of a "support role" for the other person. This doesn't usually end up very well as the "supporter" eventually is challenged on some communication or behaviors they have, which then can make them very defensive. A good mindset is that relationships are a two-way street and both, or all members have a role in the way the relationship works. A 50 - 50 approach is much more feasible. All members are there to learn new skills for their role in the family or couple. Being open and honest will reap the most benefits, but understandably, it can be difficult due to defensiveness and feelings of vulnerability.

Group Therapy (Yalom's rules)

Introduction

Group therapy is a very common way that people learn and develop important insight and skills for many different types of stresses and issues they face. There's no denying the power that groups can have on the individual. When running well, group therapy can be very empowering, often through not feeling so isolated with whatever issues are faced. Connecting and learning from others who are facing similar circumstances provides an opportunity for the individual to learn new skills, understand tried and effective techniques, and reframe their perception of their life and values. A feeling of comradery and family can be the support many needs to gain the strength to face their challenges. We are never isolated islands; we are an interconnected species that gains from relationships with others - whether just 1 person or 100 people.

How Does It Work?

We are humans, very diverse, and unique to each other. We all come to the table with different approaches to life and difficult situations. Sometimes people differ in approaches, and group therapy generally tries to accommodate all of them. Dr. Irvin D. Yalom is a psychiatrist who developed core group therapy principles that are used for any group's goals and benefits. The principles instill the guiding factors that help any group become fruitful and meaningful. Most of every group in the mental health professional setting learn and use Yalom's Principles of Group Therapy as a guide to group therapy. It's important to remember that group therapy can vary by subject and by the therapist.

The Principles of Group Therapy
The Instillation of Hope – believing one can get better with the group
Universality – sharing of experiences, thoughts, and emotions
Imparting Information – moments of educational and insightful information
Altruism – goal of helping others and benefiting from helping others
Capturing the Essence of the Family – serving as a supportive family to help specific dysregulations
Socialization Development – learning new social skills and engagement
Imitative Behaviours – role modeling and beginning to imitate positive behaviours
Interpersonal Learning – gaining insight, whether good or bad and working through preconceived notions of others in the group
Group Cohesiveness – the ability for the group to bond and support each other
Catharsis – ability to allow releasing of strong repressed emotions in a group setting
Existential Factors – learning how to be a part of something bigger than you

Table 4.3 Yalom's Group Therapy Principles

There are no absolute "rules" that need to be followed in a group setting other than universal respect for others. Group therapy can also vary in formality, from an informal 12 step meeting to a highly structured and formatted cognitive behavioral group therapy session.

What Should I Expect?

As with any new scenario, you can expect to feel nervous and intimidated on your first, even second session of group therapy. This makes sense! These are strangers, and you are about to hear and tell things that may be very private and vulnerable. Almost always, everyone in the room is feeling the same feeling, so it may be beneficial to act as you would want others to act with you during this time. This can help role model how you expect to be treated. Some people will naturally be more open than others, and that is expected. Typically, in my experience, the more open one is in a group, the more that person gets out of it. While some may simply sit in silence and listen, active participation will be encouraged, as this is the whole point of group therapy. If you are uncomfortable with groups or have some social anxiety, try individual therapy first. If you are partial to groups, group therapy can also be a more cost-effective treatment option as it generally is less expensive than individual therapy. Of course, the goal of any mental health treatment is to find what works for you! Some people flourish in group therapy; others not so much; the idea is to explore your options and opportunities to feel better.

Hypnosis

Introduction

Long misunderstood, feared by some, life-changing for others. Hypnosis generally translates to an altered level of awareness or consciousness, along with high focus and concentration. Definitions do vary as well, and of course, this is different than the hypnosis you see at circuses or magic shows, and no, hypnosis does not involve a pocket watch swinging back and forth. And yes, you are awake the entire time; falling asleep makes you unconscious and, thus, not responsive to the therapist. Hypnosis can be controversial in the mental health field because the research data doesn't have very strong evidence for its ability to help - especially compared to cognitive behavioral therapy (CBT). Hypnosis has some studies that show it can be helpful for pain, both acute and chronic. Entering into intensely relaxed states can be very useful for anxiety and stress, which is similar to mindfulness meditation.

How Does It Work?

Hypnosis works by taking the body to an ultra-relaxed state where the power of suggestions can arise. Imagine this being like taking down the walls of your castle that you are trying to protect. The walls are your defense mechanisms that rebuke any suggestions for change. This is built on a framework that humans can be resistant to change, even subconsciously. The idea of suggested new behaviors can be scary and we may be defensive against these suggestions. Once in the deep state, the therapist will then offer suggestions that are conducive to your goals and wellbeing. When the brain is in a deeply relaxed state, the walls are down, and the mind can take on these new suggestions and start to change maladaptive thinking. Sometimes, the therapist will do guided imagery, where the therapist suggests imagining calming scenes or mental images that are relaxing. Once the therapeutic suggestions are done, you are then out of the hypnosis, or deep state of relaxation.

What Should I Expect?

Hypnosis is not for everyone; either by choice or by an actual ability to do hypnosis. Studies show that how easy it is for a person to enter into hypnosis, the better the results. Those who have more difficulty getting into a state of hypnosis will obviously have less benefit if any at all. Many factors comes into play when considering how "easy" someone can enter into a hypnotic state. Some state it's how you view hypnosis (positive or negative), how well your body is able to relax itself, sleep-wake brain difficulties, and more. Roughly about 15% of people will be able to enter into hypnosis easily, while 10% find it darn near impossible, or actually impossible to do. Once again, hypnosis isn't for everyone, especially if you believe it's not going to work. Maybe it's placebo, maybe it's mindfulness with guided meditation, or it's actually what it claims to be. It is not so much that we need to know "how it works" or the "mechanics," but more, we need to focus on the results it can give people. Some people have done wonders with hypnotherapy and, thus, it can always be seen as an opportunity to try something new, with relatively little side effects. The important overarching theme, again, is that we are all unique humans who need to find our unique treatments that work.

Psychotherapy and Health Insurance

As with any treatments, health insurance covers only certain ones. Generally, health insurance likes to cover psychotherapies that are heavily researched and generally, time-limited, meaning that they average about 10-15 sessions. This includes the CBT, DBT, PET, CPT, ACT, EMDR, and, to a lesser extent, psychodynamic and couples' therapy. There are more covered, but this is just a note that health insurance may not cover certain psychotherapies you may be interested in. This isn't to say that those non-covered psychotherapies are not useful or effective, it's just how health insurance is covering certain ones over other ones.

Adjunctive and Complementary Therapies

We never want to just "manage symptoms" for our mental health. We are unique individuals who have purpose, meaning, and individuality. The essence of "wellness" and "wellbeing" require treating the whole picture, and complementary and alternative therapies can help complete that picture. Complementary and alternative medicine therapies (CAM) are products or practices that generally are not a part of the general mainstream medical treatment for any given condition. They are "enhancers" and give uniqueness and wellness to the individual. CAM works very well in mental health. Most of the CAM therapies are attending to the basics of our human nature and giving them "tune-ups." Integrative Medicine is a bright new field of medicine that uses the standards of medical care plus the use of CAM therapies. We are continually learning more and more about the different CAM therapies and their effects on wellbeing

Supplements

Supplements are a product that replaces, helps to compensate, or enhances the body. It's important to know that we live in a world where supplements or natural products can help out tremendously but also hurt us more than conventional treatments. The word "natural" gets thrown into so much, but "natural" doesn't mean "healthy." Think of it, poison ivy is natural, but not healthy for us. Alcohol is legal and natural; simply let some fruit ferment, but that does not mean that it is "natural = healthy" for us to consume

Below you will find the most researched and best supplements for mental health. Please note that supplements are not FDA regulated, which means that the product you buy may state it has a certain amount of the supplement but may not have that amount.

St. John's Wort

- A long-known supplement to help depression and anxiety, St. John's Wort increases serotonin, which is the brain chemical that helps calm anxiety and relieves depression
- Interestingly enough, people want to try St. John's Wort for "natural" purposes, but it typically has the same side effects as conventional antidepressants, such as nausea and sexual dysfunction
- One uniqueness of St. John's Wort is its interactions with other medications. St. John's Wort interacts with a lot of different types of medications, often leading to safety issues. Combining St. John's Wort with another antidepressant can cause serotonin syndrome rather quickly. Caution should always be sought.

s-adenosylmethionine (SAM-e)

- This is a natural chemical in our body
- The supplement helps with depression and anxiety
- Most research shows that it does help with depression and anxiety with an important factor that most people don't have any side effects
- It should be noted that SAM-e helps with depression in some studies, but it can worsen symptoms in bipolar disorder

Omega 3

- Of the supplements, Omega 3s have been studied the most for mental health conditions
- There seems to be some evidence that Omega 3s help protect the brain along with reducing inflammation in the brain, which can contribute to relieving depression and anxiety
- Interesting, most research states that to get the mental health benefits

from Omega 3s, you need to take much higher dosages than conventional Omega 3 dosages (normally to help your heart)
- The biggest part of Omega 3s, EPA, needs to be over 1000mg to get a decent effect
- Side effects most commonly associated with Omega 3s are acid reflux and indigestion

5-HTP

- 5-HTP is a chemical that comes from tryptophan, which is found in meats we eat
- 5-HTP is an amino acid (protein) that eventually becomes serotonin. Serotonin is that brain chemical that helps with feeling well, reducing depression and anxiety
- 5-HTP should not be taken with a prescribed antidepressant or St. John's Wort as it may cause serotonin syndrome

Folic Acid

- Folic Acid is a B vitamin (B9)
- Folic Acid has substantial research showing it to enhance antidepressant medication for depression and anxiety
- Research indicates that it doesn't work as a stand-alone treatment

Chamomile

- Long used as a tea for calming and relaxing properties
- The mechanism of action isn't well understood, but studies show that chamomile can help generalized anxiety as much as conventional medications

Valerian

- Valerian is derived from the root of the flower, *Valeriana officinalis*.
- Valerian has been studied and is known to help with anxiety and insomnia
- We don't quite understand how Valerian works, but we suppose it works by increasing the brain chemical GABA
- It can cause stomach upset

Magnesium

- A natural element, magnesium is a known supplement for blood pressure issues
- Magnesium can be sedating, which can help with insomnia and anxiety
- Magnesium in high doses is used to control seizures in pregnant women (normal anti-seizure medications would hurt the fetus)
- Magnesium has side effects, such as diarrhea, nausea, and vomiting

Exercise

We all know that exercise is an important component to try and incorporate into our lives. The more and more we study exercising, the more we learn of its benefits. The body was not built to be in the world it is in today. Watching TV – sitting at an office -lounging; these are all creature comforts of the modern era. Unfortunately, our bodies don't like this, they like to move, and when they don't, your body can warn you with poor mental health feelings. Interestingly enough, most people believe that exercise means going to the gym or running endless miles. Nothing could be further from the truth. Exercise is simply being mobile and moving around. Walking, hiking, mall shopping, simply moving your arms, and more is exercise. Exercise is what you make it, and when you create your unique exercise plan makes it more motivating and engaging because it's on your terms, not some other person's idea of what "exercise" is.

Some of the benefits of exercise include brain growth. Exercise not only works out your muscles and heart, but it also works out your brain. Exercise makes your brain more resilient to changes and stressors. It does this by increasing an important brain ingredient, brain-derived neurotrophic factor (BDNF), which is a bodyguard for your brain along with a construction crew, building new parts of your brain to help it function better. Exercise also increases the brain chemicals serotonin, dopamine, and norepinephrine. There is plenty of research that points to the boosting power of exercise on serotonin, our feeling good, and anxiety-reducing brain chemicals. Intense exercise can increase norepinephrine, which helps with concentration and focus. Dopamine is released after completing each exercise. That feeling of pleasure and motivation can be intense after an exercise. This helps motivate you to exercise more and more. The famous "runner's high" is your natural opioid (painkilling) chemical, endorphins, released in your brain while exercising. And guess what, you get it when you exercise in any way, it doesn't have to be running. It is released more during intense exercise. Exercise reduces stress hormones cortisol and adrenaline. These are hormones that contribute to much of the health diseases we see today, and lowering these stress hormones means you can handle more in your life. Exercise is known to improve sleep. We are sleeping creatures, spending upwards of 1/3 of our lives sleeping. Exercise can improve sleep by helping you expend those stress hormones that keep you up and wreak havoc on your sleep quality. Exercise can also increase blood flow to your brain, especially to the parts of the brain that help regulate your mood and reduce anxiety and stress. All these critical factors help with regulating your mood, decreasing stress, and motiving you to take on more challenges.

There is an evolutionary pattern to these functions. Sitting around and isolating tells your brain that you are not gaining the resources you need to survive. Start to move around (exercise), and your brain rewards you with increased energy, calming, focus, feeling good, and motivation to keep it up. It's always an advantage to tap into the benefits that our brain naturally gives us.

Diet

A healthy diet is a part of our lives that is usually very difficult to obtain and maintain. Our body has a preference for natural foods because it is the most efficiently used for energy, but our minds might take us elsewhere. In today's modern society, we are a sugar, fat, and processed food-craved people. Interestingly, foods that are normal for our body's chemistry are viewed as "healthy food." This shows how normalized our society has got to eat foods that are not natural to our bodies. Often, I tell people we shouldn't eat "healthy," we should eat "normal." This means choosing foods that our body is the most geared towards using for energy and wellbeing and not foods that just taste good but wreak havoc on our body. Our mental health community faces big consequences when diet and nutrition become erratic. Some medications are prone to metabolic issues, making diet and nutrition even more important. We all have a good idea of what a decent diet looks like, and it's not the fad diets we all see. Plant-based foods are very beneficial to our mental health, along with our heart health. Avoidance of processed foods is important as the ingredients from these foods are nutrient deprived and may even cause inflammation, which as some research indicates, can contribute to depression. Sugars and carbohydrates have been especially noted to cause issues with mood, especially depression, anxiety, and sleep issues. There isn't necessarily a "right" diet. Focusing on foods that are natural and reduced in processing is key. Foods that are natural tend to have much more nutrients than foods that are processed. The most highly researched and evidenced-based diet is the Mediterranean Diet, which consists of many fruits, vegetables along with fish and other low-fat meats.

Here's the truth: you want to find your own diet that is consistent with being nutritious and benefiting your own mental health. Can't make a full commitment? Remember that small changes can lead to bigger results. Try making one meal a day a "healthy" meal and go from there.

Socializing

We are a social creature. Our relationships and need to belong with others are fundamental to what it means to be human. More and more, our modern society is allowing people to be more isolated and disconnected from humanity than ever before. Research is showing that this has a huge impact on our mental health. Think about it....you could walk around New York City, with all those thousands, if not, millions of people you see and never say one word to one person. That tells you how incredibly isolated we can become. The benefits of connecting with others include learning about others, which creates an appreciation and mature connection with others. People in isolation never fair well with their mental health. The only people who generally feel "okay" with complete isolation are those with a schizoid personality disorder. Historically, we were much more connected with others. When in contact with others, we learn how to self-regulate our thoughts and feelings. Think about talking to your friend about some jealousy you have, and they keep you in check with your feelings. This helps you to regulate what is a normal feeling versus a detrimental feeling that is unjustified. Our family gives us roots into who we are. No one on earth can be your biological parents, biological cousins, and so forth. Something to note is that healthy relationships are key. There are many family relationships that are very detrimental to a member's mental health, so take everything with caution. Relating and connecting with others is crucial for a harmonic society. Have you ever wondered why soldiers in the Middle East or Israel have much less PTSD than those soldiers in the U.S? Many other countries' general population go through war with their soldiers, creating a common experience. In the U.S., the general population is generally disconnected from war, and the U.S soldiers who come back from war come into a nation where nobody understands them. This disconnect makes their symptoms start to exhibit

10

SUBSTANCE USE AND ADDICTION

"I have absolutely no pleasure in the stimulants in which I sometimes so madly indulge. It has not been in the pursuit of pleasure that I have periled life and reputation and reason. It has been in the desperate attempt to escape from torturing memories, a sense of insupportable loneliness, and impending doom."
-Edgar Allan Poe

Addiction How it Works

What is addiction? Is it only to substances? Is it a disease? Is there such a thing as an "addictive" personality? These are widespread questions I hear regarding addiction. Mental illness has its stigma, but addiction takes a whole new level of stigma in society because it is viewed as a choice, weakness, moral issue, and more. It can "create criminals, breaks up families, turns the most loving person into the evilest person," and so on. Addiction can wreak havoc and ruin just about anyone's life. But we must always try to remember that behind every "addict" is a human. No one shoots out of the womb going, "I really want to grow up and be a drug addict." A lot of times, people with addiction have extensive trauma, has family who uses substances, and more. It has always been my experience that learning how the brain and addiction works helps us to connect with those struggling with addiction and also provide that insight that anyone is prone to addiction, it could be heroin, money, sex, fitness, eating, smoking, buying cars, or anything else that taps into the system we are about to learn about.

The brain is a funny thing. In many ways, unpredictable, in other ways, very systematic and rule-based. The brain evolved bottom-up (which makes sense) with our primal, animalistic system being the bottom and most archaic. The newest (and what makes us human) is the top neocortex (literally meaning "new brain"), which aids in decision making and social abilities. The older the system, the stronger it typically is. Thus, our emotions, anger, fear, and lust part of the brain can override our new part of the brain that helps with controlling those emotions. It was built this way for survival. Your brain is primed to immediately be afraid and run (or fight) if you are getting attacked or potentially dying. This old and strong system, called the limbic system, also contains the area where we learn, get rewarded, and even get some of the best feelings we ever have. When we experience something fun, or that tastes good, or feels good, etc., we are blasted with the brain chemical dopamine in this old strong reward part of the brain. This teaches us to try and keep doing that action because it feels good. Your brain has "learned" that this experience feels good, which then makes your brain "motivated" to seek it out again. The stronger the dopamine (feeling good) you get, the more easily learned, engrained, and motivated you get to seek it out again. This is how addiction occurs, and it's when this system becomes out of tune.

But how do we keep control of this usually? Well, that brand new (well not so new) part of your brain? That neocortex? It contains the prefrontal cortex, which is your impulse control and decision making part of the brain. For example, you see a big cake in the kitchen. Your limbic system goes wild, starts shooting dopamine into your limbic system, which is saying to you, "you love this cake, this cake is so amazing, do you remember how great this cake is? It will make you so happy, and you will love being happy." Your prefrontal cortex then comes in and says to you, "whoa! Hold on, slow down the limbic system. Remember that your cholesterol is pretty high, and you need to lose about ten more pounds. You said before that this was a good goal to have and in the long run will make you happier, healthier, and live longer."

This interplay between these two systems is constantly happening in our everyday lives. The decision to buy Starbucks, the decision to study for that exam, the decision to go to the gym, etc. Some people have a stronger prefrontal cortex, some of a stronger limbic system. By default, the limbic system is older and thus can overrun the prefrontal cortex pretty easily if it feels threatened (think anxiety, being scared, pressured, timelines, and of course, life-threatening situations).

Geez, too much science stuff here. Let's look at an example that we can all relate also, Snickers bar

Imagine you have never had chocolate before. Don't even know what it is. A friend gives you your first Snickers bar. You open it. Your brain is looking at this and going, "okay, I guess I'll try it." You take your first bite. BOOM! A rush of dopamine into the limbic system. It tastes fantastic, and you feel happier; you feel motivated to take another bite. Your brain is happy. It has just learned that this so-called Snickers bar is delicious, makes you happy, and should be sought after again. You are in the supermarket a week later waiting to pay for those healthy vegetables you just picked up. You see in the candy aisle a box of Snicker bars. Your brain automatically shoots dopamine into that limbic system. "Oh yes, that Snickers is so good, remember how good it was? How happy you got instantly? Let's do the behavior of buying a bar right now," and then you do. All that talking was dopamine in the limbic system. It's motivating for you to buy the bar so you can feel good again.

You are starting to like Snickers bars. Your body is learning more and more that Snickers bars make you feel good. The more you indulge in them, the more your brain learns and learns. Guess what, you just formed a habit.

Soon, you are sitting at home in your chair watching TV. You merely "think" of a Snickers bar. Your brain gives you a dopamine boost (a craving) to motivate you to get up and "seek" that Snickers bar. This means you have to get up and drive to the store and get one. You see how the habit and the seeking behavior gets more and more over time and with more indulging.

Now replace Snickers bar with _____. Gambling? Sex? Meth? Alcohol? Fast food? Gym? Shopping?

It doesn't matter what it is. The brain works the same in how it forms the addiction. The more powerful the substance or behavior is, the more you learn, and the more ingrained it gets.

This leads to dominant seeking behaviors, which is what can lead to so much turmoil - stealing, prostitution, lying, divorce, loss of children, whatever it may be. Substances that are abused, either illicitly or legally, almost always use dopamine in the limbic system. The powerful substances we know of attach to the receptors in the brain and essentially "release the floodgates" of these powerful brain chemicals. Now that we have a little understanding of how addiction works. We can move a step further and learn about the most commonly used substances seen in addiction and see the specific ways they work in the brain.

Alcohol and Benzodiazepines

Alcohol is an incredible substance. It infiltrates so many more areas of the body than traditional substances. It also is different in how it affects the brain. Most substances that are used target maybe 1-2, rarely three different types of brain chemicals to get their effect. For example, marijuana mimics the brain chemical endocannabinoid and also a little bit of brain chemical dopamine. Another example? Heroin mimics the brain chemical in the opiate system and also targets dopamine.

Alcohol targets six brain chemicals. Alcohol reaches far and hits hard in the brain. Some brain chemicals are hit harder than others, so when treatment is done, we tend to focus more on those brain chemicals for better results. In a nutshell, these are the brain chemicals affected:

- **Serotonin** -increases when drinking alcohol, drops when coming off alcohol
- **GABA** -increases when drinking alcohol, drops when coming off alcohol
- **Opiates** - increases at high amounts of alcohol, drops when coming off alcohol
- **Dopamine** - increases at height amounts of alcohol, drops when coming off alcohol
- **Endocannabinoid** -increases while drinking, dropping when coming off alcohol
- **Glutamate** -steadily increases with heavy, everyday drinking

Let's break these down to make sense of how alcohol does what it does:

Serotonin: this one makes sense; when you drink alcohol, it has a powerful antidepressant and antianxiety effect. We can thank the increase in serotonin for that. The only unfortunate side is that it has "rebound effect," meaning that once the alcohol wears off, you are not just back to normal levels of serotonin, you are now lower than you were before = more depression, more anxiety

Opiates and Dopamine: when you increase your drinking (say binge drinking) in one night, you begin to tap into the opiate and dopamine system. This is what "numbs" you physically and emotionally. Put in dopamine, and you now are feeling euphoric, giggly, more sociable, etc. Not only that, but the dopamine surge now has deeply rewarded you and is not the main motivator for you to drink to that level again

Side Note: learn about Naltrexone and how it works with these brain chemicals to reduce binge drinking

Endocannabinoid: wait, what? Isn't that the system that marijuana targets? Yes, there is some research that points to the endocannabinoid system being activated by alcohol, mostly involving the digestion and appetite of the person. Hungry anyone?

GABA and Glutamate: These two are very important brain chemicals when looking at alcohol because they are the basis for its use and why alcohol has such nasty side effects. GABA is that calming brain chemical. GABA reduces anxiety, promotes relaxation, but also keeps the nerves and brain cells in check from being revved up to high, which can cause seizures and heart issues. Can you guess what alcohol dramatically increases when you drink it? You got it! GABA. Now, glutamate is a brain chemical that does the opposite. It excites your body, gets the nerves going, makes the brain and heart fire more. Our bodies are made to have GABA and glutamate do a balancing act. GABA keeps glutamate in check, glutamate keeps GABA in check. When one is high, the other is going to try and increase to counter it (why can't we all just be friends?!). We know when you drink alcohol, you immediately get calm, but can you remember the next day? Have you ever felt more anxious? Tense? More irritable? That's due to the excess glutamate that has increased in order to balance with the GABA rush from last night's night out drinking. When alcohol becomes daily and heavy, glutamate is constantly fighting the GABA rushes you are giving it.

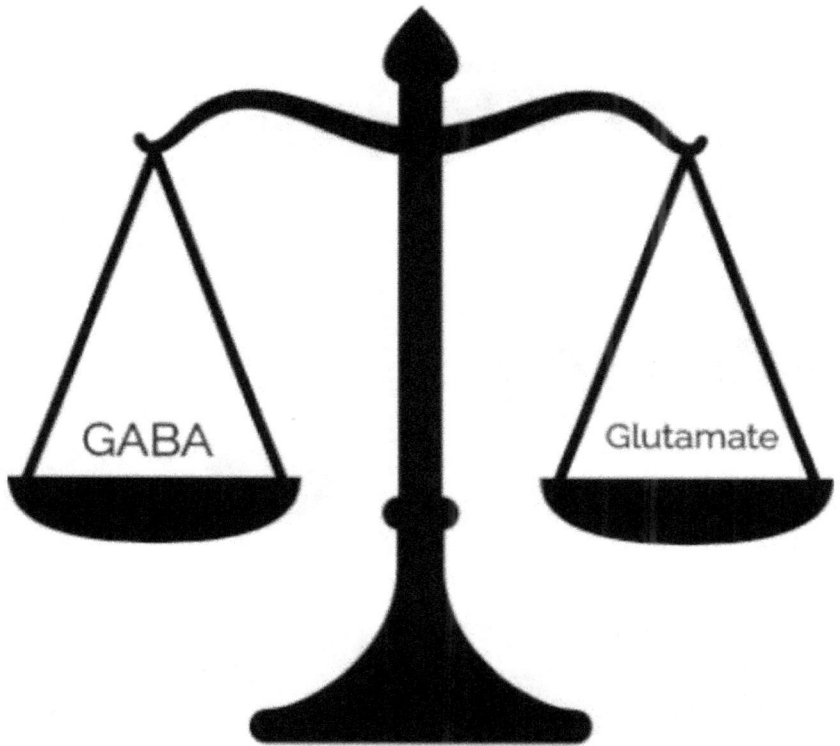

Figure 5.1 GABA and Glutamate play a balancing act in your body on a normal everyday basis

It wants desperately to fight it and balance out. Now, you take away alcohol, and you just released the roof on the glutamate. It skyrockets like the Old Faithful geyser at Yellowstone National Park. The competitor didn't just weaken; it's completely gone.

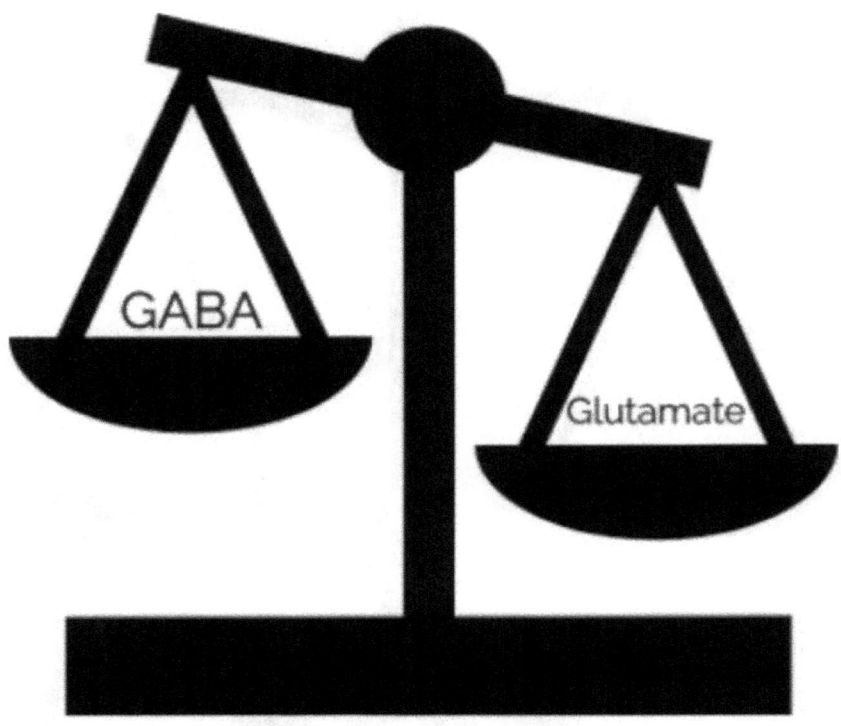

Figure 5.2 When you drink alcohol, your body gets a surge of GABA (anxiety relief)

This leads to glutamate surging in your body, causing muscle twitches, agitation, confusion, and worse, seizures and heart issues. This is withdrawal, and it is incredibly dangerous. When a person who uses alcohol daily tries to stop, they risk their life. You hear of people who use alcohol saying that they need it "to be normal," they are simply doing the job of the GABA system (which has run out and not working) and trying to balance it out with the excess glutamate.

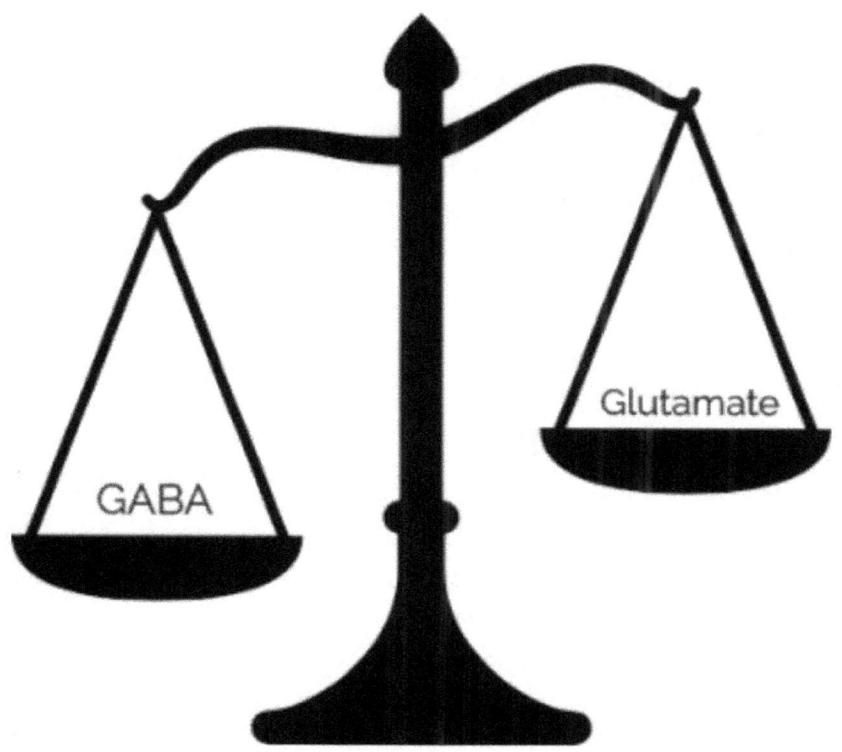

Figure 5.3 With GABA surging from alcohol, glutamate (excitatory) has to counter this surge by having its own surge.

Alcohol and benzodiazepine withdrawal are by far, the deadliest of the substances to withdraw from. The risk of seizures, heart rhythm abnormalities, and brain damage can and is lethal. Unfortunately, both alcohol and benzodiazepines are generally seen as "safer" substances than others. Alcohol, for all intents and purposes, is one of the most consumed beverages in the world and is advertised to be "fun," "socially outgoing," "letting loose," and so on. Benzodiazepines are, for the most part, prescribed by a doctor or prescriber. This can give the false allusion that benzodiazepines are safe and "healthy" to use simply because they are prescribed to you from a trusted health professional. Both of these perceptions are very detrimental to anyone trying to acknowledge a substance issue, let alone, being able to abstain from these substances. Later in this book when we discuss treatments, you'll see that one of the most powerful tools in abstaining from any substance is completely avoiding being near it. This sometimes means ditching old drug buddies or your bar friends, but in general, avoidance and creation of a new "normal" is crucial. This is very difficult when alcohol is everywhere from the TV, grocery store, family reunions, concerts, billboards, and so many more.

A note on benzodiazepines

Benzodiazepines (Ativan, Valium, Klonopin, Xanax, Librium, etc.) have been an increasingly problematic issue in the addiction field. Benzodiazepines were first noted for their ability to help anxiety with the advent of Librium, which is considered the first benzodiazepine created. We see benzodiazepines used in many areas of the healthcare field, from alcohol and benzodiazepine detoxification to emergency seizure medication, anxiety, and insomnia. One of the biggest problems with benzodiazepines is that they work well. I mean, they work VERY well. You pop a benzodiazepine, and anxiety and panic just shrivel away. To have such power in a pill to get rid of anxiety and typically within 15 minutes of taking, it is truly astonishing to anyone who suffers from anxiety.

Benzodiazepines and alcohol work very similarly. Both have the main target of GABA, that brain chemical that helps our body relax. Like alcohol, benzodiazepines build a tolerance very quickly. This is where people get in trouble. In all honesty, benzodiazepines were never made to be a "maintenance" drug, meaning to be taken over months and years. They were designs for short term emergency relief of extreme anxiety and agitation. This is because of the tolerance building and guess what, tolerance building happens in every brain. This is not one of those, "oh, but I don't have an addictive personality" type excuses. We all build a tolerance. So, you may start with 0.5mg of Ativan. Whoa, that works well! You start taking that 0.5mg of Ativan daily to quell the anxiety. By week 2, that anxiety is creeping in again. "Darn, maybe I'll take 1mg of Ativan. Aww, that's nice." This goes on and on, and by the time some months go by, you may be needing to take 4-5mg of Ativan a day just to get the same effect of the original 0.5mg in the beginning. This is tolerance building, and unfortunately, it creeps in on unsuspecting people who are merely taking medications from their prescriber and are trying to help their anxiety issue. Now comes the tough part. Coming off them. Your body is very used to having these medications keep that GABA chemical up to get rid of anxiety. Now, with the medication gone, we get a big surge of that anxiety-causing glutamate. This is called "rebound anxiety," and for anyone who has had an issue with benzodiazepines, they know what this means. Some people will immediately go into panic attacks, and some will start to seek out the benzodiazepine in the streets. Some will need to go through detoxification to ween off the medication.

There is growing evidence that benzodiazepines dramatically increase the risk of Alzheimer's, a type of dementia. Some data shows that taking a benzodiazepine for 3-6 months can raise your risk for Alzheimer's by 32% and if it goes for 6 months and longer, up to 84% increased risk. There is ample evidence that benzodiazepines cause anterograde amnesia, which is a fancy way of saying that you cannot remember any event or partially an event when on a benzodiazepine. Whatever the case is, benzodiazepines have some considerable risks and should be cautiously prescribed if prescribed at all. In California, where I practice, prescribers are to look at the narcotics databases to see if patients are taking a benzodiazepine, opioid, or muscle relaxer. There are then limitations and liabilities if found that a patient is taking one, two, or all of the above. Benzodiazepines do have their place in the healthcare field and are wonderful agents in seizures, extreme agitation, and short term treatment for panic attacks until an antidepressant kicks in. Caution must always be considered.

Opiates and Heroin

As we speak, there is an opiate crisis in the United States. So much so that overdoses now are the number one accidental death; previously and for years, it was car accidents. A part of this tragedy comes straight from our dearly trusted medical industry. When the article from the Joint Commission on pain was introduced in 2001, there was a paradigm shift in the medical field. Noted pain was to be considered the "fifth vital sign" (the others being heart rate, respiration rate, blood pressure, and temperature), the goal was to get the pain to a "0" on a 0-10 pain scale. Was this necessary? The call to treat pain was a major factor that needed to be dealt with. For years, many people, especially those with chronic pain, would needlessly suffer because of very conservative prescribing by most physicians. Once the Joint Commission's report came out, physicians were not only loosening up on treating pain, major hospital systems, and practice guidelines put tremendous pressure on prescribers to get the pain to a "0." What we have now is a paradigm that has swung the other way. Now, statistics show that 80% of new heroin users started on opiate prescription pills, most for a legitimate pain issue. Of the opiate pills, OxyContin is one of the worst culprits in abuse numbers. In 2019, the makers of OxyContin, Purdue Pharma, have lawsuits in virtually every state for the dramatic rise and tragedy of opiate overdoses. The jump from opiate medications to heroin use is super-efficient for anybody in any class. The relative easiness to obtain along with cheap cost of heroin gives the craving mind the perfect way to get satisfied. One of the biggest shocks with the opiate epidemic is how widespread between socioeconomic parties it is. Many of the middle class and wealthy class have equally been hit hard by the opiate epidemic. Grandmothers, parents, no one is safe from the opiate epidemic.

One important factor for anybody to know about opiate overdoses is that the majority of overdoses and deaths result from the person relapsing after an extended period of time. As someone uses opiates, tolerance builds and builds. By the time they decide they want to quit, they may be taking 40mg - 100mg of oxycodone daily, if not more. Now, say this person decides to try to quit. They are successful, go through the detox, and remain off opiates for 4 months. Now, a big stressor. A breakup, or a death. This person decides they need a break from these terrible emotions and decides to use the one thing they know will take the emotional pain away, opiates. So, he goes and takes that 40mg of oxycodone because that's what he was using when he stopped. Next step? Overdose and possibly death. This person's body is not used to the high levels of opiates anymore. The brain has re-regulated and becomes sensitive to opiates again. By taking this 40mg of oxycodone, it hits his brain with tremendous force, leading to sedation and eventually, respiratory arrest. The other way a lot of overdoses and deaths are occurring is by taking opiates with another substance at the same time. Gabapentin (Neurontin), generally very safe and effective pain medication, has been used for years in pain disorders and anxiety disorders. With the opiate crisis, there has been a discovery of using opiates with gabapentin to get high and this substantially contributing to the toxic effects that kill people. This has become such a factor in overdoses that the Drug and Enforcement Agency (DEA) is now looking at reclassifying gabapentin to make it more restrictive. This again puts a well-known, generally safe pain medication out of reach for those who need it.

Opiates would be much safer if the opiate system in our body weren't so friendly with other brain systems. What do I mean by this? The opiate system, when activated, activates a whole array of systems in the brain. Of these systems, the opiate system is best buddies with the GABA system. GABA, if you remember, is the brain chemical that relaxes your body, takes away anxiety, and alleviates fear. When the opiate system is activated by an opiate pill or heroin, GABA is also released in large quantities. This is what leads to the calming effect that many people who take opiates crave. Couple this with some release of dopamine to make you feel even better and (most importantly) learn and become motivated to seek out this experience again and you have the recipe for opiate misuse. Part of what grabs so many unexpected people into opiate use is underlying trauma, depression, anxiety, or general stress that gets alleviated by taking an opiate. This to a naive body that isn't used to substance alteration is a big shock and is quickly learned that this is what you do in order to get rid of all this stress, anxiety, shame, and guilt you never knew could go away. Another conundrum of opiates is that when you take heroin or opiate medications, your own natural bodily opiates (endorphins) stop being made. The brain shuts off the production of endorphins because it's saying, "well, we have plenty of opiate in our system; we don't need to make anymore." This leads to the person stopping the opiate, not only feeling pain (whether emotional or physical) but feeling pain at a much worse level than before taking opiates. This reinforces the need to keep taking the opiate in order to not feel worse than before.

It should be noted that alcohol and opiates have a lot of cross-addiction. What does this mean? People who misuse alcohol are at a higher propensity to abuse opiates and vice versa. This is due to the opiate - GABA interplay between the two substances. You drink alcohol, you get GABA, which then releases endorphins (opiates). You take opiates, you get opiate, which then releases GABA. This can be important to know in case you are in recovery from alcohol and are prescribed an opiate or vice versa. Because opiates are taken to numb pain and tough emotions, when a person is coming off of opiates, it is almost unbearable to manage day to day stressors. Typically, you'll see that more opiates are taken during more stressful times. This leads to the body learning that when the going gets tough, the more you need numbing. Now, when off opiates, when the going gets tough, you feel much worse. This is the same for most substances but is particularly true with opiates.

What does the future look like? There is much push for prescribers, like me, to aggressively treat opiate addiction. As for those with pain disorders? There needs to be a rebalancing of the paradigm bell as there are those with legitimate pain issues that are withheld vital medications that can ease the pain. There is new research that is looking at unconventional pain relievers such as cannabidiol oil (CBD) for pain relief. Unlike marijuana with TCH (the psychoactive part of marijuana), CBD does not have any psychoactive part to it and is being researched for pain management with moderate to good results. This isn't a cure-all for the opiate crisis. The damage and colossal epidemic will take years to quell down and will likely be one of the costliest substance abuse epidemics in our time.

Methamphetamine and Stimulants

Methamphetamine (meth), or as a patient told me once, "the poor man's coffee," is an incredibly powerful stimulant, cheap to make, highly toxic, and highly addicting. The process of making meth involved pseudoephedrine (Sudafed), a common anti-congesting medication. The toxic chemicals used to extract and make meth are very toxic, and it is said that making one pound of meth makes 5 pounds of toxic waste. This doesn't even mention the dangers of meth labs involving explosions. Meth is smoked, eaten, injected, put in the rectum, and probably many more ways I've never heard of before. When taken, the brain surges with high, toxic amounts of noradrenaline (adrenaline) and dopamine. The noradrenaline gives intense energy, racing mind, feelings of invincibility, where dopamine gives more euphoria. The dopamine also is the addiction part of the brain, so the brain learns very quickly that meth "feels good" so you want to "take meth again." Meth causes all sorts of problems for individuals taking it. Frequently involved with the law, meth makes you highly impulsive, so doing more drugs, stealing, robbing, breaking into cars and such can be done without your brain even having a chance to contemplate the consequences. This increased energy and euphoria can also lead to impulsive sex acts and sex with multiple partners. It is no secret that prostitutes tend to use meth as a way to escape the psychological terror involved in their profession, but also to be able to make the body able to "work" even though her mind doesn't want to. Historically, prostitution saw a lot of opiate use (morphine) in order to disrupt ovulation and prevent pregnancy. Meth also tends to be seen a lot in the construction world as it gives the energy needed for those grueling 10-12 hours of hard labor. Coming off of meth is usually a 2-3 day deal called a "crash". While generally with a safe withdrawal, there is a feeling of the flu coupled with hours and hours of sleep. When awoken, the meth is typically cleared, and the repeated behaviors begin again. Meth (and prescribed stimulants) have a high propensity to cause psychosis. This is due to the intense increase of dopamine from the substance. You can see paranoia, delusions, grandiose "I am God" thoughts, and hallucinations. This, with the intense levels of energy, can lead to very dangerous situations of violence and trauma and should be taken with caution. If you have a loved one who uses meth, try to avoid "enraging" topics while they are in the throes of meth intoxication. It's hard to help your loved one when you yourself are hurt.

Prescription stimulants have been around since 1944 with the advent of methylphenidate (Ritalin). Used for Attention Deficit Hyperactivity Disorder (ADHD), prescribed stimulants have been the gold standard for helping children with attention and hyperactivity do well. Prescribed stimulants are highly sought medications. They are incredibly popular in colleges and universities as they are seen as a "study drug" that helps with studying for exams. Stimulants can be highly abused, especially those of the amphetamine class (Adderall, Dexedrine, Vyvanse). Ritalin and other stimulants can be abused but not have the powerful effects of the amphetamine class. The reason has to do with how the medications work on the brain. Stimulants work by increasing noradrenaline to help focus and concentration in the prefrontal cortex (decision making, impulse control part). It also increases dopamine incidentally, helping with learning and motivation. These abused medications mimic methamphetamine and have the same effects seen in meth. There are contradictions in the mental health field with regards to stimulants and ADHD. There is research that points to the overuse of stimulants and abuse, while there is research showing that there are many children undiagnosed with ADHD. There is also dramatic debate regarding "adult-onset" ADHD, where ADHD appears in adulthood rather than in childhood like most ADHD. Research, in general, shows that what appears to be "adult-onset" ADHD is typically something else manifesting, be it depression, anxiety, bipolar, traumatic brain injury, or other manifestations. It is nonetheless weekly I get a person telling me they have ADHD that started at age 30, to which further investigation is always needed.

When considering putting your child on stimulants, always try to rule out other distracting factors related to attention issues or hyperactivity. We live in one of the most distracting environments ever known, with technology and everyone trying to grab your attention. I always advise parents to look around the house. Are there massive amounts of toys? This can be overstimulating. Are there electronics like iPads or phones they play with? This can wreak havoc on attention span as games are geared to be an intense and fast pace experience. This isn't handy when they need to read "Huckleberry Finn" for their book report. Is there bullying? Is there a possible trauma occurring? You can't focus on your education when you are scared of your livelihood. If these factors are looked at, then there are scales and tests that can be performed to see if the ADHD-like symptoms are consistent across time and space (a critical factor in diagnosing ADHD). There are even computer programs (Quotient Computer Test of QOT) that take 15-20 minutes and helps analyze many aspects of ADHD through many mini-tests. These options should be sought before any stimulant is introduced to your child.

Another consideration if you have an adolescent, say 15-25 years old, who has a sudden onset of psychosis (paranoia, voices, delusions, etc.), always consider the possibility of drug-induced psychosis. Many times, we can get a high school teen who is very psychotic, treat them with antipsychotics, only to have them completely clear up and go on in life, learning from their mistake of abusing Adderall. Now, some do abuse a stimulant and "unlock" a predisposed brain to illnesses like schizophrenia, bipolar, and schizoaffective disorder. The important thing to understand is that the initial treatment is the same — treatment with antipsychotics — because the parts of the brain and chemicals involved are the same between the two. Psychosis is very common with stimulants and meth, but also with other substances, such as marijuana, "spice" (synthetic marijuana), bath salts, and other substances.

Marijuana

Oh, marijuana. I wonder how many people picked up this book and went straight to this section to see what I have to say about marijuana. Marijuana is as old as old can be. There is evidence of our ancient ancestors either eating or smoking cannabis plants and utilizing cannabis for all sorts of ailments. The "high" that comes from marijuana comes from a chemical in marijuana called tetrahydrocannabinol (THC). This psychoactive substance gives you the calmness, relaxed, giddy, elated feeling that is known. Marijuana has gone through a lot in the past 30-40 years. From a hardcore drug offense (some places gave life sentences!) to having a multitude of states either decriminalize or actually allow the recreational use of marijuana is somewhat of a miracle, and also room for lots of confusion about marijuana.

Is it good? Is it bad? I'm okay to use it, but you aren't? What is the answer? Well, the answer we all enjoy is the one I'll give, "it's complicated." For one, marijuana today is not the same marijuana from 1969 that mommy and daddy smoked. With technology and learning about the growth of marijuana, lots of marijuana today is intensely stronger (more THC) than ever before. This changes how you look at marijuana. We are seeing much more psychosis related to heavy marijuana use. Sadly, I admit that ten years ago, when I would assess for substance use, if the person said, "I use marijuana," my general reaction was, "okay, what else are you using and how much?" I couldn't really be bothered by marijuana. I wasn't seeing people on the inpatient unit or in inpatient detox there for strictly marijuana use. This has changed dramatically. The potency of THC greatly increases the risk of psychosis, especially with heavy daily use. It used to be that marijuana was balanced in a way with cannabinoid oil (CBD) and THC as CBD has antipsychotic properties. Today's THC's levels decimate the effects of the CBD in marijuana, leading to this increased risk of psychosis.

Interestingly enough, research is seeing different effects from the two main types of marijuana, Indica, and Sativa. Indica is known for its body relaxation and calming sensation, while Sativa is more understood to give a more "head high," energy with calmness type high. Research is demonstrating that Indica has a high likelihood of memory loss or disturbances, while Sativa has a high likelihood of psychosis. To make matters worse, people are now concentrating THC even more than before. This butane hash oil (BHO) or "dabs" is an oil that is highly concentrated with THC and has an incredible risk factor for psychosis and memory issues.

So, with the understanding coming from the research and observed cases over the past years, marijuana should be taken as a serious drug. One that can cause impairments and detrimental effects on the brain. There is an illusion that if something is legal, that means it's safe, and this couldn't be farther from the truth. Just look at alcohol and cigarettes, which kills millions each year. So much of the time I hear that marijuana has no side effects, but the medications I prescribe have side effects. Marijuana does have side effects — sedation, difficulty concentrating, erectile dysfunction, low sperm county, energy level fluctuations, and not to mention lung damage if smoked, and more. When marijuana is stopped, there can be a rebound effect where anxiety is more intense than before. These side effects though, are generally just offset by the power of the effect and the quickness it relieves anxiety, pain, or whatever is being managed with it. The other argument I typically hear is that marijuana is "natural." So is poison ivy and cockroaches, both are things I don't partake in because of its "natural-ishness." We must always be wary when people use the "natural" word in any product. They are tying the word "natural" to mean "safe" or "meant for us," and this simply is not the case. There are plenty of examples of "natural" products that have ended up hurting a lot of people in history. Funny enough, sometimes I point out that lithium (a mood stabilizer used in bipolar disorder) is a natural salt, found all over the earth, yet this example is typically discounted in some way or the other by some interesting reasoning. Here's the theme to that story: people will come up with lots of reasons why something they like is okay, and definitely will come up with reasons why something they don't like is awful and terrible. In reality, it's probably a little of A and B.

As time moves forward and the legalization of recreational marijuana becomes more widespread, we will see the outcomes of marijuana in the general public. I'm open to finding new ways that marijuana can benefit people, especially with the promising literature on CBD with opiate addiction. For some, marijuana may be as benign as drinking soda (only in moderation, of course), and for others, it may have devastating effects. The problem we face is that we usually don't know the latter until much devastation has occurred. A more important conversation, either with your loved one or yourself, if you use marijuana, is to examine your reasons for marijuana. Are they because of data and empirical data? Is it because of an underlying reason, such as anxiety or depression? What bias might I have with marijuana? All these questions can shape the way we see a substance and may even cloud our judgment to the actual benefit to risk factors. Always keep your health in mind.

Cocaine and Crack

Cocaine and its cheaper cousin crack are not as popular as it was in the 1980s and 1990s. Part of this has to do with international fighting over the cocaine sources in South America and the difficulty of crossing borders and with the advent of new meth production techniques. Meth, you can buy cold or sinus medicine in the pharmacy, cook up meth in a hotel room, then sell it and get an instant profit. All without crossing borders and dealing with drug lords (in different countries). Still, we do see the cocaine and crack use in the United States. Cocaine has been used for years as a pain reliever and even for hysteria by people like Sigmund Freud in the late 1800s. Cocaine as an abused drug became popular in disco 1970s and the 1980s as it was seen as a party drug. Typically reserved for the rich due to the price, people would get high from snorting cocaine within 5-15 minutes, which would then dissipate after 30 minutes to 90 minutes and then be either met with the decision to do more (take another "bump" or "raise") or hit a downer effect (depression). Tolerance to cocaine is built rapidly, so maintaining a high can be difficult for a long time. Typically, if a person wants to keep their high going, they will use absorbent amounts. Most people cannot afford to keep this habit up, and most will stop after a "night binge." The effects of cocaine are euphoria, numbness, intense happiness, and anxiety/agitation. Cocaine is still used mostly as a "party drug" today, and the main route is through snorting.

Crack cocaine is the drug dealer's dream and everyone else's nightmare. To take expensive cocaine and break it down to a smokable freebase crack that is not only cheaper but hits your brain harder leads to one of the worst drug epidemics in the United States. Crack's cheap price and the instant high were devastating to inner cities and the poor. Crack, typically smoked, but can be injected, gives an immediate 5-10 minute high. The quickness of the high leads to the user having to constantly take more and more, consuming every part of their day to keep the high going. Crack gives you euphoria and intense feelings of happiness and invincibility, but it also leads to extreme agitation, paranoia, and skyrocketing blood pressure and heart rate. *Parasitosis* is the delusional feeling that you are infested with bugs and is seen in both crack cocaine and methamphetamine use. Long term use of cocaine and crack leads to "crack lung" and "crack heart failure," both of which are a result of the toxins destroying tissues in your body. Crack is not as common as it used to be but is still seen largely in inner cities and with homeless populations.

Cocaine and crack are neurologically messy. By dramatically increasing dopamine, serotonin, and noradrenaline all at the same time, you get this mishmash of feelings that overwork those systems, making it difficult to treat. Dopamine is the main brain chemical that is the troublemaker with cocaine. Big spikes in dopamine lead to the euphoria and feelings of invincibility seen in crack and cocaine, but it also contributes highly to the paranoia and psychosis that can occur. Noradrenaline leads to stimulating and energy boost but is the main driver of agitation and aggression. All three of these brain chemicals make dramatic drops when the cocaine is stopped, leading to the intense "cravings" that is so commonly seen and experienced in order to try and rebalance the depletions. These drops also lead to the crash that is felt after cocaine, which is typically depression, irritability, and lethargy. Even though there have been drops in cocaine and crack use, the general pattern seems to exist still today, where cocaine is generally seen in the club scene and typically with the rich, famous, politically connected, while crack cocaine ravages the poor in inner cities, both causing erratic havoc because of the powerful change's cocaine causes in the brain.

Nicotine and Tobacco

Nicotine and tobacco are some of the most common and deadly substance dependencies in the world. 1 in 5 Americans use tobacco or nicotine products. Around 1 billion people smoke in the world according to the World Health Organization (WHO). Tobacco kills more than 3 million people per year. We all understand the harms of cigarettes and tobacco products, but why do we tend to bypass the importance of these harms in the mental health field? The word *intensity* comes to mind. Nicotine and tobacco don't alter your brain and change your behaviors drastically, then say alcohol, heroin, marijuana, et cetera. There doesn't exist a crime of "nicotine driving" or killing a person because of "nicotine intoxication." In this way, nicotine and tobacco subtle effects, ease of use, and the immediate result (the nicotine effect) are what makes nicotine and tobacco so dangerous and insidious. Like many substances, the number of people using nicotine is typically deemed by the culture. There are areas in the United States that have higher smoking and tobacco rates than other areas. Utah and California have the least nicotine and tobacco use at 8% and 11%, respectively. This is partially due to Utah being a highly Mormon population, which bans the use of nicotine and tobacco, while California's low use is due to massive media campaigns and laws barring smoking and nicotine in certain private and public areas (restaurants, within schools, out front of stores, bars). The highest rates of nicotine and tobacco use are in the South, where Kentucky and West Virginia top the list at both 25%, or 1 in 4. Once again, the culture of these areas tends to have more relaxed laws on tobacco and nicotine use along with these states being the highest producers of tobacco crops and tobacco products.

"So, I heard that nicotine is so addictive that smoking one cigarette can make you addicted." Not really. As a matter of fact, most people will tell you that the first time they tried a cigarette, they felt nauseated and had a massive headache. I know this from experience, but with trying chewing tobacco for the first and last time. It indeed takes time to become a full-fledged nicotine user. Many people smoke only when they drink alcohol, and that is because alcohol hits all the brain chemicals except for two, acetylcholine and noradrenaline. Guess what brain chemicals nicotine hits? Acetylcholine and noradrenaline. Thus, completing the puzzle and affecting all brain chemicals to give the fullest effect of mind high. Acetylcholine is useful for memory and cognition speed while noradrenaline gives energy while also giving increased focus and concentration. The other brain chemical that is involved, and is in all other addictions, is dopamine. Dopamine, again, is that brain chemical responsible for how addiction forms, or strong learning patterns. It gives you pleasure, you learn of that pleasure, and then become motivated to seek out that pleasure more. This is what gives nicotine the addictive edge that grips so many people. Nicotine, as a chemical, is generally not as toxic as we might believe. Nicotine does alter brain chemicals, and yes, there is nicotine toxicity, but we are generally unsure of long term wear and tear on the brain from nicotine. What hurts and kills people is the byproducts in tobacco and chemicals in nicotine products.

A note of vaporizers or "vaping"

A relatively new method of smoking nicotine has become widespread in the United States and across the world. Vaping uses a battery-powered heater to instantly heat "e-juice" or "e-liquid," which is typically glycol or glycerine based solutions. They will typically contain nicotine and flavorings of all sorts. Is vaping safer than smoking tobacco? At this time, yes, there are much fewer toxic chemicals in "e-juice" than in cigarettes. Does that mean it's healthy? No. Just as the legalization of recreational marijuana, there is a perception that when something is legal and less dangerous than other substances, that makes it okay to consume. While much less harmful than cigarettes, vaping still has nicotine, which is highly addictive and can lead to dependency. Inhaling anything into your lungs except for oxygen, water, and natural secretions can be highly irritating to the lungs, leading to increased congestion. Admittedly, in 2019, we simply don't have enough evidence to point to any direct dangers other than the nicotine argument. That may be good or bad for the future. We may learn that vaping is rather harmless; we may learn with many consequences that vaping is very detrimental to health.

Nicotine, smoking, and mental illness

We know that people with mental illness have a higher propensity to use substances to self-cope. Smoking and nicotine rates are very high in the mental health community. The specific brain chemicals that nicotine raises, acetylcholine, noradrenaline, and dopamine, can give immediate benefits to those with mental illness who typically are deficient in these brain chemicals. Smoking and nicotine use are especially high in psychotic disorders, and even more so specifically in schizophrenia. The brain's thought disorganization, difficulty concentrating, and difficulty showing emotion is a strong feature in schizophrenia. Smoking raises the correct chemicals that give temporary relief to those specific symptoms. You will see that it will clear their thoughts, become less disorganized, and increase the ability to express emotion. There is also evidence that nicotine can mitigate some of the side effects we see with antipsychotic medications.

Other Notable Substances

Bath Salts

One of the more visible and prominent substances right now is the designer drug *bath salts*, which are not actually bath salts, they merely resemble bath salts. Instead, this designer drug is a potent stimulant, similar to methamphetamine. Smoked, snorted, injected, or ingested, bath salts lead to a 5-hour high that increases energy, pleasurable feelings, and euphoria. Often combined with alcohol, the combination enhances each other and so often used in social settings. Bath salts are very well known for their terrible adverse reactions. Headache, nausea, hallucinations, and panic attacks are only the beginning. Being a stimulant, it can cause intense paranoia and panic attacks. There are some reports of heart attacks and impulsive suicides from bath salts. As of 2012, the main psychoactive ingredient, mephedrone, is banned, but some skirting around drug laws occur when labelers but "not for human consumption" on the labels. There are no tests to detect bath salts as of 2019.

Synthetic Marijuana "Spice"

Spice made its wave of use in the late 2000s. I remember working in a drug and alcohol residential program for parolees and people being high and paranoid, and we couldn't even detect spice nor even recognize what it was. We would find all these K2 (one of the spice brands) packets everywhere that stated it was incense, which was allowed in our facility. Spice is synthetic marijuana that mimics THC, the psychoactive chemical in marijuana. Although effects are similar to marijuana, spice is highly unpredictable. The potency of synthetic THC is many times higher than regular marijuana, and there are numerous cases I have seen and is known countrywide of panic attacks, heart-pounding, nausea, vomiting. It gets worse. Spice is well documented for causing intense paranoia, confusion, coordination issues, and even seizures with possible death. The psychosis rates are very high with spice because THC makes a person prone to psychosis. Not only that, but regular marijuana contains CBD (cannabidiol), which has antipsychotic properties. Spice does not have CBD, thus allowing the THC to wreak havoc unopposed. Spice is not detectable in most drug tests, and a specialized (and very expensive) test is needed to detect spice. Banning spice has been arduous, and spice is still seen in the United States today, especially with teenagers.

Anabolic Steroids

Anabolic steroids remain a stable substance used in the sports and fitness world. We use anabolic steroids in the medical field for a variety of illnesses, typically involving the immune system, but for the sake of this book, we will be geared to the illicit use of anabolic steroids. Steroids kick your body in energy-producing, muscle gaining mode. This is typically at the sacrifice of allowing your body to rest and regulate. Like flooring the gas pedal on your car, the parts start to wear down faster. Steroids are notorious for its sexual side effects of infertility, reduced testicular size, and erectile dysfunction. Because testosterone levels are involved with prostate health, steroids can cause an enlargement of the prostate and even prostate cancer. Muscle breakdown from overuse can occur and cause kidney failure (rhabdomyolysis), acne and skin changes can occur, high blood pressure, high cholesterol, heart failure, heart wave issues, heart attacks, and sudden death can also occur. For the purposes of this book, steroids can cause a person to have massive mood swings, typically with an overarching agitation and irritability. Sometimes called "roid rage," violent behavior is seen and even psychosis with paranoia.

Interestingly, steroid use and suicide seem to correlate. Sad cases involving professional wrestlers killing their family and then themselves have occurred and with contribution from steroids. Even with such adverse effects, steroids remain prevalent and common, especially in competitive environments. Steroids can be found in blood lab work but are specialized tests and are not conducted regularly unless suspected.

Inhalants

Inhalants (or huffing) involves inhaling chemical vapors in order to get an instantaneous high that is very temporary (a few minutes). Typically, the short high leads the person to repeatedly keep taking hits in order to maintain the high, causing havoc on the brain. Most commonly used items are "dust off" (used to clean the dust off electronics), paint thinners, gasoline, white-out, permanent markers, glue, lighter fluid, spray paints, hair spray, and more. With so many options and ease of use, huffing can be hard to control. Huffing essentially takes the chemical straight to the brain and deprives it of oxygen and absorbs the toxic chemicals causing slowing of the brain, euphoria, dizziness, visual disturbances, and speech changes. Long term use can lead to extensive brain damage and have psychotic features. Can people die with inhalants? Absolutely! Seizures can occur from such disruptions to the brain, which can cause sudden death. I know an individual who was huffing and suffered a seizure and passed away. Inhalants are typically seen as "fun," "temporary," and "harmless." Huffing is more seen in younger populations, especially in the teenage years.

MDMA, Ecstasy, and GHB

MDMA, Ecstasy, and GHB are "club" drugs that generally have the same effect of euphoria, increased sociability, and increased sex drive. All last about 5-6 hours (perfect for clubbing). MDMA and Ecstasy work by drastically increasing the brain chemicals serotonin, norepinephrine, and dopamine, leading to increased energy and euphoria. GHB hits an exciting GHB part of the brain leading to increased energy while drastically increasing the brain chemical GABA, which is calming and causes euphoria. GHB can be used as a "date rape" drug because of this combination. What you will see is that the brain will "turn off" memory formation and awareness from the GABA increase, but the body and brain will remain awake because of the excitatory GHB part of the brain being activated (same effects happen with caffeine and alcohol mixtures). GHB also reduces the ability of the body to eliminate alcohol, which is also used in the club and party scenes. This leads to many overdoses and death seen with GHB. Overdoses are common with club drugs and are typically related to heart and respiratory-related (heart attacks, breathing problems), as well as convulsions and seizures. Typically, after a binge with these club drugs, a person may feel depressed, anxious, irritable, and craving more. GHB is a predominant drug in the gay scene. MDMA/ecstasy is generally predominant in younger people, especially those in the "rave" or club scene. Tests are available, but typically not used as the club drugs are metabolized and leave the body rather quickly.

Abused Medications

We are aware of the more commonly abused prescription medications like opioids (Norco, Percocet, Vicodin, Fentanyl, and more), stimulants (Adderall, Ritalin, Vyvanse, and more), and benzodiazepines (Ativan, Valium, Xanax, and Klonopin). There are previous sections above that discuss these three types.

Here, I wanted to share some other commonly abused medications that should be made aware. The first is *bupropion (Wellbutrin)*, a common antidepressant that raises the brain chemicals dopamine and noradrenaline. While a very low potential for abuse when taken orally (only prescribed way to do so), crushed and snorted, bupropion gives an effect similar to cocaine. While bupropion is still a very good drug to use in depression, we are seeing it being abused in high-risk environments, such as jails/prisons and addiction treatment centers. Another prescription medication, *gabapentin (Neurontin)*, is common nerve pain, anti-seizure, and anti-anxiety medications. Generally, low side effects and very low abuse potential, gabapentin has been used without any discretion for years and has been off the radar as abusable. Gabapentin, though, when combined with other drugs, such as opioids, can enhance the high from those drugs. Some studies have shown that up to 1 in 4 overdoses from heroin had very high levels of gabapentin involved as well. It's too bad this medication is being used in this way as it will certainly be met with laws and controlling policies, and I have personally seen gabapentin do wonder for people with chronic pain and anxiety. The other medication to be aware of is *dextromethorphan*, or *DXM*, and is commonly found in over the counter cough medicines. Taken orally at dosages 3-75 times the recommended dosage amount, the person experiences euphoria, dissociation, dilated pupils, and some with hallucinations, muscle spasms, and high heart rate. This "space out" drug is very commonly seen in the high school and college settings. Coming off of DXM can present with depression, irritability, anxiety, and flu-like symptoms.

Gambling

Gambling is a section I wanted to include in this chapter, as it is a common addiction that has absolutely devastating effects. Addictive learning patterns are very common with many different types of mediums, for some its substances, for some, it's fitness, for others maybe being the center of attention, but the basic parts and chemicals in the brain that learn these addictive behaviors are the same. What makes gambling dangerous is that Casinos and gambling venues have spent every ounce of energy into creating worlds where this addictive part of our brains is inundated. They are literally geared to tap into this part of the brain and to get you hooked. It's not a secret that Casinos pay (very well) top psychologists in the world to research and create the reward patterns for all their machines and game tables. Free drinks loosen inhibitions, make you feel good that this is worth investing, the mere lights actually create happy feelings. Gambling machines are programmed with a variable reward pattern, which has been heavily researched to keep people engaged without giving too much away. Rewards are random, always have, always will. There is no "luck" or "knowing" the outcome of these machines. BUT, you may invest five times and get a little reward, then maybe three times, but then maybe 25 times and so on. The psychology behind variable reward patterns is to make it unpredictable but to also give little rewards (which psychologists have research amount of time) in order to keep the person thinking that indeed there is a big reward about to happen. If there were no little rewards, then the person would get angry and go. Give too many little rewards, and the casino loses out.

Gambling also works on another part of our behaviors, investment. Casinos make gambling enticing because it's so little investment. What are 5 or 10 cents to have a little fun? And there's the hook. You start off with a small investment, but with little unpredictable rewards, you become more invested. Before you know it, you are inherently invested in the game. Simply leaving is hard because you lost all the investment, staying and putting in more will surely have a big payout; it's just around the corner. This idea of fairness and investment is crucial to us as humans as we should feel that if we invest in things like relationships, learning skills, or investing time into being creative, that there should be a level of reward or benefit. Gambling completely screws with that part of our human nature as gambling doesn't play fair but is actually robbing you. Gambling plays into our strong tendency to pattern seek, which is trying to find patterns when there is chaos or unpredictability. Once again, an archaic mechanism of creating order and meaning, gambling taps right into this, often making people feel that they can learn the pattern or that they know how to "cheat" the game and win big.

When talking to people with gambling addiction, you will see that there is a sense of being out of control. Even more interesting, much research into gamblers shows that there is a sort of "trance" that they enter when engaged in the game. The constant surge of dopamine that is helping you learn this addictive pattern also gives your massive pleasure, so this "trance" or "slot machine zone" creates a world where all problems and personal struggles go away. There are also studies that point to gamblers (and many other humans) being absolutely terrible at estimating winnings versus losses. How many people have you heard saying they won big in Las Vegas and, of course, every time they ever played in Vegas? It may not be a deceitful or denial intention to "lie" about the losses; their brain probably doesn't have the correct amounts counted. Indeed, this adds to the potential for gamblers to be shocked when they see their bank accounts go to 0 because, in their minds, they had been winning.

Gambling has absolutely terrible consequences. Going into debt, losing the house, losing all your retirement are common stories in gambling addiction. My father has worked in the funeral industry for many years and managed several mortuaries in the Las Vegas area, and it was no surprise when there would be a surge of elderly suicide victims with gambling addiction, typically around 7-14 days into the month, right when the social security check would run out.

Treatment can be very difficult for gambling addiction. The ingrained pattern in that primitive part of the brain is very strong and very rigid. You never truly unlearn addictive patterns; your goal is to learn new patterns that override the addictive pattern. To do this is to learn activities that are more rewarding than the addictive behavior. Cognitive Behavioural Therapy (CBT) is the treatment of choice as it challenges the distorted thoughts regarding gambling and puts into perspective the actual losses and consequences of gambling, while also building new coping skills. Group therapy has been seen as beneficial to gambling addiction. Groups, such as Gamblers Anonymous, create a special time to express your challenges while learning from others on techniques they have used to stop gambling. Like substance abuse, one of the best techniques to stop gambling addiction is to simply avoid it, avoid the building, avoid the friends at the casino. For some, this may be changing the car route to avoid seeing the casinos to full-blown moving to a town where casinos are illegal. The decision on intensity is yours and unique to your circumstances.

11

SUBSTANCE USE AND ADDICTION TREATMENT

"To be free from suffering, be free from attachments"
–The Buddha

Addiction Treatment

Treatment for addiction varies tremendously. The field of addiction is vast and is generally complicated with different methodologies and conflicting ideas of how to best treat people with addiction. This further gets into how people view addiction.. Is it a disease? Is it a moral issue? Is it a learned behavior? Is it due to underlying mental illness? For years, addiction and mental health were seen as two different arenas. You still see this today. You have no idea how many times I have to decide if somebody is "substance abuse" or "mental illness" for entrance into a program. Each addiction theory will have its own position on what the right treatment is. In general, addiction treatment centers have soared in the past 20 years. Unfortunately, many private and public health insurance coverages have not, leading to a huge disparity in treatment options for most people with addiction. This leads most addicted people and families having to make huge financial decisions and sacrifices to get any reputable addiction treatment done. Unfortunately, this is in addition to the varied quality amongst each addiction treatment facility; some of which are barely maintaining any accreditation, if any. Addiction treatment also varies in approach, with some being very relaxed to ones that involve intense structure and harsh tactics. Unfortunately, the more money you pay, the more relaxed treatment you get in most scenarios.

Deciding to seek treatment for addiction is very tough. You are putting yourself in a position that will not only be extremely uncomfortable but also taking away the one thing you always did when you felt stressed. There are many options in addiction treatment and trying to navigate the system to find the right treatment for yourself, or your loved one is daunting. One aspect to consider is the level of treatment you are willing to engage in. Old school thought would be to have you immediately go to a 30 day residential, 100% in treatment at all times, setting. The idea behind this is that you want to literally squash the addiction out of the person. When addiction treatment is sought, there are typically very high emotions. Anxiety and worry may be common, but so may hurt and aggression towards the addiction. Extreme emotions can lead to extreme choices. The truth is that many people with addiction can successfully treat their addiction with less intensive treatment options. A general statement to live by is "the least invasive that is also the safest." What does this mean? Well, research shows that people with addiction can fair well and actually have more investment in treatment if it is incorporated into their everyday life. Safety, of course, is if there is a withdrawal component. Benzodiazepines and alcohol withdrawal are by far the most harmful of all drug detox, which can be lethal.

Expenses can be a large factor in choosing addiction treatment. Indeed, some addiction treatment may cost upwards of $60,000 a month for treatment. Private insurance may cover a portion of this, but it's typically minimal and with many restrictions. One aspect to investigate with any treatment center is the professionals that are on staff. Do they have a physician? A clinical psychologist? Therapists? Nurses? Counselors? Why pay $60,000 for a treatment facility that is nothing more than a hotel with a glorified 12 step program (which is free)? I've personally always advocated for treatment that is non-12 step, or at least not mainly based on 12 step. Why? It has nothing to do with 12 steps per se. 12 step treatment (Alcoholics Anonymous, Narcotics Anonymous, and more) is a group treatment for addiction, and are almost in every city and free for anyone to use. Why pay for a treatment that you can readily get for free? If someone is going to pay for addiction treatment, especially in the tens of thousands of dollars, you might as well pay for addiction treatment that actually costs money to receive. 12 steps can easily be added to the treatment for free by going to groups in the community. Addiction treatment for some families can literally lead them into financial destruction, especially when the person with addiction repeatedly goes back due to relapsing. This is why it's important to know that research shows that people with addictions can manage well on an outpatient basis that is more cost-effective.

Does the person with addiction want treatment? This is always very hard to gauge as many families and loved ones put unintended pressure on people with addiction to accept treatment. Unless the person actually wants to get well, addiction treatment may end in disappointments, which then reinforces the person to use substances again as "this is just who I am" or "there is no fixing me." A person with addiction absolutely needs to have a say into the type of treatment they are to receive. This can be hard as some will want only very minimal, if any treatment at all, but in the end, it isn't about us, it's about their buy in to actually go through the difficult treatment. Giving some choice and preference to treatment allows the person to feel that they are invested in the treatment choice, which increases motivation and engagement. Do you remember ever being forced to do something as a child? Maybe going to church? Or having to do your chores when your favorite TV show was on? Your level of engagement was minimal at best, let alone the resentment and lack of motivation to actually go through with the task. Sure, these were "good" and "healthy" tasks for us to do, but the point is not that it's good for us. It is very important to know that addiction, by its nature, is very resistant to "punishment." That is because the awful feelings that come from punishment are easily remedied by the substance itself, making punishment useless and more harmful. The point is that no one will engage in something naturally, nor be intrinsically motivated to take care of themselves unless they feel they have some choice in the matter. I cannot tell you how many difficult discussions I have had with families stressing that forcing their loved one to go to this ritzy residential addiction center was not going to end well because the person felt pressured and didn't want treatment. Almost always, the person would use substances again. Addiction is tough, and seeking treatment is even tougher. It's always important to remember that humans like to be respected, and to someone with an addiction who already feels that they are out of control, this respect of choosing their path to recovery is more potent for them than the average person.

Alcohol and Benzodiazepine Treatment

Alcohol treatment is one of the most sought after treatments in the addiction field. Alcohol is readily available and has a huge cultural component in society. Benzodiazepines are an anti-anxiety medication that is used for anxiety disorders. As far as the brain is concerned, alcohol and benzodiazepines are the same things. Both raise the calming brain chemical, GABA, while also raising other brain chemicals, such as dopamine, the main brain chemical involved in addiction. Alcohol and benzodiazepine treatment almost always involves detoxification in a facility that is equipped to handle this dangerous detox. Indeed, alcohol and benzodiazepine withdrawal are the deadliest of any substance withdrawal. This is because alcohol and benzodiazepines raise GABA, which inversely blocks a brain chemical called glutamate, which is an excitatory brain chemical (more energy). When you stop alcohol or benzodiazepines, this brain chemical glutamate skyrockets like a geyser at Yellowstone National Park. High glutamate causes seizures, shaking, agitation, and heart rhythm distresses that can be lethal. You will rarely see a methamphetamine withdrawal in an intensive care unit, nor cocaine, but alcohol and benzodiazepine withdrawal make a lot of people end up in an intensive care unit, on the fringes of death.

Alcohol and benzodiazepine treatment are typically called detoxification, or "detox." This is a medical treatment, not a therapeutic treatment. Therapy and counseling will come later when the person is deemed safe to participate. Alcohol and benzodiazepine treatment will contain the use of (sounds odd) benzodiazepines. To reduce the high levels of the brain chemical glutamate, the person takes benzodiazepines to keep the brain from getting too overactive. This overtime is decreased to allow the brain to readjust itself to normal brain chemical levels. Even though this detoxification treatment can be done in outpatient, treatment centers, you want to make sure they have proper medical personnel there handling the detoxification. Hospitals are the best setting for this. Clinical detoxification will involve an assessment called the Clinical Institute Withdrawal Assessment scale (CIWA) (Figure 6.1). This scale measures the detox symptoms based on severity and then medicates those symptoms accordingly. The goal is to provide comfort, but also to prevent any serious medical harm, such as a seizure or heart rhythm issue.

Once a person has detoxed from the withdrawal period, they can begin to engage in treatment that aims to understand and tackle the addiction head-on. In many ways, the best therapy treatment for alcoholism and benzodiazepine abuse is as unique as the person who is using them. Generally, a therapy that involves cognitive behavioral therapy, along with the development of new coping skills, can help tremendously. Learning about your association with the substance can be beneficial, as well.

Clinical Institute Withdrawal Assessment Scale for Alcohol, Revised (CIWA-Ar)

Nausea and Vomiting
0 – No nausea or vomiting
1
2
3
4 – Intermittent nausea with dry heaves
5
6
7 – Constant nausea, frequent dry heaves and vomiting

Paroxysmal Sweats
0 – No sweat visible
1 – Barely perceptible sweating, palms moist
2
3
4 – Beads of sweat obvious on forehead
5
6
7 – Drenching sweats

Agitation
0 – Normal activity
1 – Somewhat more than normal activity
2
3
4 – Moderate fidgety and restless
5
6
7 – Paces back and forth during most of the interview or constantly thrashes about

Visual Disturbances
0 – Not present
1 – Very mild photosensitivity
2 – Mild photosensitivity
3 – Moderate photosensitivity
4 – Moderately severe visual hallucinations
5 – Severe visual hallucinations
6 – Extreme severe visual hallucinations
7 – Continuous visual hallucinations

Tremor
0 – No tremor
1 – Not visible, but can be felt at finger tips
2
3
4 – Moderate when patient's hands extended
5
6
7 – Severe, even with arms not extended

Tactile Disturbances
0 – None
1 – Very mild paraesthesias
2 – Mild paraesthesias
3 – Moderate paraesthesias
4 – Moderately severe hallucinations
5 – Severe hallucinations
6 – Extremely severe hallucinations
7 – Continuous hallucinations

Headache
0 – Not present
1 – Very mild
2 – Mild
3 – Moderate
4 – Moderately severe
5 – Severe
6 – Very severe
7 – Extremely severe

Auditory Disturbances
0 – Not present
1 – Very mild harshness or ability to frighten
2 – Mild harshness or ability to frighten
3 – Moderate harshness or ability to frighten
4 – Moderately severe hallucinations
5 – Severe hallucinations
6 – Extremely severe hallucinations
7 – Continuous hallucinations

Orientation and Clouding of the Sensorium
0 – Oriented and can do serial additions
1 – Cannot do serial additions
2 – Disoriented for date but not more than 2 calendar days
3 – Disoriented for date by more than 2 calendar days
4 – Disoriented for place/person

Cumulative scoring

Cumulative score	Approach
0 – 8	No medication needed
9 – 14	Medication is optional
15 – 20	Definitely needs medication
>20	Increased risk of complications

Figure 6.1 CIWA Scale for Alcohol Withdrawal

Symptoms of Alcohol Withdrawal Syndrome

Time of Appearance after Cessation of Alcohol Use	Symptoms
6 to 12 hours	Minor withdrawal symptoms: insomnia, tremors, anxiety, gastrointestinal upset, headache, diaphoresis, palpitations, anorexia, nausea, tachycardia, hypertension
12 to 24 hours	Alcoholic hallucinosis: visual, auditory, or tactile hallucinations
24 to 48 hours	Withdrawal seizures: generalized tonic-clonic seizures
48 to 72 hours	Alcohol withdrawal delirium (delirium tremens): hallucinations (predominately visual), disorientation, agitation, diaphoresis

Figure 6.2 Effect of time lapse and alcohol withdrawal symptoms

At times, some people who have successfully come off of alcohol or benzodiazepines take medications that help to prevent relapse. While there isn't such medication for benzodiazepines, for alcohol, there are three main types.

Naltrexone (Revia)– a medication used to reduce the number of drinks during a single session (example – drinking two drinks instead of 8 drinks). It works by blocking the brain chemical dopamine, which rises higher and higher as you drink alcohol, further leading to addiction

Acamprosate (Campral)– used to prevent cravings of alcohol and, thus, any desire to consume alcohol. This works by stabilizing the cravings when the body feels like it may withdrawal from alcohol

Disulfiram (Antabuse)– used to avoid any alcohol consumption. If the consumption of alcohol occurs, the body will violently vomit. This works by stopping the enzyme that breaks down alcohol from working. This leaves your body filled with alcohol that makes it feel toxic, thus activating the vomit response to get rid of it.

While there is no one-shot solution for alcohol and benzodiazepine treatment, many people have successfully come off of both of them and have gone on to lead very successful lives. The goal for any addiction treatment is to always find what will work for you best.

Opioids and Heroin Treatment

We face an opioid epidemic. Much like the crack epidemic of the 1980s, the opioid epidemic has devastated many people and their loved ones. In 2017 alone, 47,000 deaths were attributed to opioid overdoses. This has been magnified with the addition of Fentanyl, an opioid that is 100 times stronger than morphine. A nice fact is that the strongest opioid in the world is actually our own, beta-endorphins. Fentanyl is an illegally marketed drug hitting the streets hard and can be so strong that police officers and other first responders have been known to overdose on it by simply inhaling some of it by accident. Treatment for opioids has, thus, exploded with many options becoming available. Many decisions are needed when seeking treatment for opioids due to the array of options.

Some questions to ponder are:

1. Do I need to detox?
2. Do I need to detox and then continue taking maintenance opioid medications?
3. What other resources do I need in place to not go back to using opioids again?

Although incredibly miserable and uncomfortable, opioid withdrawal does not kill you. It's always important to remember that withdrawal symptoms are always the opposite of what the drug's effects are. So, imagine a painkiller withdrawal. Knowing that the withdrawal will be the opposite effect, you essentially are experiencing a lot of pain during withdrawal. Withdrawal treatment thus, involves controlling these withdrawal symptoms.

Detoxification typically lasts 4 - 7 days and typically is an inpatient event. Medications used during detoxification include the following:

- **Muscle Relaxer** - muscles start to spasm and create a lot of pain when detoxing off of opioids. Muscle relaxers help take the edge off this pain
- **Anti-Diarrhea** - opioids make you constipated. This is because of opioids numb your intestines, essentially slowing them down or turning them off. When you stop an opioid, the intestines go into hyperdrive, causing diarrhea
- **Anti-Nausea** - opioid detoxification can cause stomach upset, which is caused by the hyperactive digestive system
- **Anti-Anxiety** - when someone takes an opioid, it inadvertently hits the brain chemical GABA (anti-anxiety). When you stop an opioid, you are then low on GABA, causing anxiety, irritability, and agitation
- **Pain Reliever** - of course, opioid withdrawals will be painful. A pain reliever is crucial during detoxification to help the person remain comfortable. Typically used is Ibuprofen 800mg or Tylenol 500 - 1000mg.
- **Suboxone/Subutex** - Suboxone contains two medications – (1) *buprenorphine* and (2) *naloxone*. Subutex contains only buprenorphine.

1. **Buprenorphine** is a stable opiate that hits the same receptors as heroin and opiate medications. It is "weaker," so you don't get a "high." It also doesn't get any stronger effect when increasing the dosages, which makes it less abusable and dependent
2. **Naloxone (Narcan)** is an opiate "blocker." When injected into the muscle or bloodstream, this can save a person's life from opiate overdose. When it is absorbed through the tongue (sublingual) or stomach, the effects are less. Naloxone taken in Suboxone works by blocking the effects of opiate abuse. For example, someone takes Suboxone and then wants to get "high," so they inject heroin. Naloxone will block the effects of heroin, thus teaching the person that they cannot get high from heroin or another abused opiates

Opioid detoxification is measured by severity using the Clinical Opiate Withdrawal Scale (COWS) (Figure 6.3). This scale measures the severity of each symptom of opioid withdrawal. This COWS score then informs the healthcare professionals how severe the detoxification is and how to medicate appropriately. Opioid maintenance, or sometimes called Medications Assisted Therapy (MAT), is another option for people with opioid addiction. MAT is controversial in the addiction world. In the theories of 12 step (AA/NA) and other schools of thought in abstinence recovery, MAT is seen as one drug addiction replacing another drug addiction. Indeed, the treatments in MAT are almost always opioids (with the exception of Naltrexone) and are used in lieu of the abused opioids. In a perfect world, yes, we wouldn't want people dependent on a medication to help with their opioid addiction, but we do not live in a perfect world. The goal of MAT is to provide maintenance medications that decrease cravings and doesn't have any mental or physical long term effects (no "highs"). This, of course, is drastically different than the previous behavior of abusing opioids to get a "high" and at the cost of their physical and mental health, along with not being able to function in everyday society. Many people on MAT live productive lives, able to work, be a part of a family, and doing so in a sober way (not being "high"). To each is their own, and I respect anyone's journey that is safe and effective. We must be able to see that a person on a MAT who is functioning in everyday life and being productive is incredibly more optimal than being in the throes of opioid cravings and abusing. It's not fair to ourselves to use black and white thinking to such complexities in life, and that's to ourselves and others.

APPENDIX 1
Clinical Opiate Withdrawal Scale

For each item, circle the number that best describes the patient's signs or symptom. Rate on just the apparent relationship to opiate withdrawal. For example, if heart rate is increased because the patient was jogging just prior to assessment, the increase pulse rate would not add to the score.

Patient's Name:____________________	Date and Time ___/___/___:______
Reason for this assessment:____________________	
Resting Pulse Rate: _________beats/minute *Measured after patient is sitting or lying for one minute* 0 pulse rate 80 or below 1 pulse rate 81-100 2 pulse rate 101-120 4 pulse rate greater than 120	**GI Upset**: *over last 1/2 hour* 0 no GI symptoms 1 stomach cramps 2 nausea or loose stool 3 vomiting or diarrhea 5 multiple episodes of diarrhea or vomiting
Sweating: *over past 1/2 hour not accounted for by room temperature or patient activity.* 0 no report of chills or flushing 1 subjective report of chills or flushing 2 flushed or observable moistness on face 3 beads of sweat on brow or face 4 sweat streaming off face	**Tremor** *observation of outstretched hands* 0 no tremor 1 tremor can be felt, but not observed 2 slight tremor observable 4 gross tremor or muscle twitching
Restlessness *Observation during assessment* 0 able to sit still 1 reports difficulty sitting still, but is able to do so 3 frequent shifting or extraneous movements of legs/arms 5 unable to sit still for more than a few seconds	**Yawning** *Observation during assessment* 0 no yawning 1 yawning once or twice during assessment 2 yawning three or more times during assessment 4 yawning several times/minute
Pupil size 0 pupils pinned or normal size for room light 1 pupils possibly larger than normal for room light 2 pupils moderately dilated 5 pupils so dilated that only the rim of the iris is visible	**Anxiety or Irritability** 0 none 1 patient reports increasing irritability or anxiousness 2 patient obviously irritable or anxious 4 patient so irritable or anxious that participation in the assessment is difficult
Bone or Joint aches *If patient was having pain previously, only the additional component attributed to opiates withdrawal is scored* 0 not present 1 mild diffuse discomfort 2 patient reports severe diffuse aching of joints/muscles 4 patient is rubbing joints or muscles and is unable to sit still because of discomfort	**Gooseflesh skin** 0 skin is smooth 3 piloerrection of skin can be felt or hairs standing up on arms 5 prominent piloerrection
Runny nose or tearing *Not accounted for by cold symptoms or allergies* 0 not present 1 nasal stuffiness or unusually moist eyes 2 nose running or tearing 4 nose constantly running or tears streaming down cheeks	Total Score ______ The total score is the sum of all 11 items Initials of person completing assessment: ______

Score: 5-12 = mild; 13-24 = moderate; 25-36 = moderately severe; more than 36 = severe withdrawal

This version may be copied and used clinically.

Source: Wesson, D. R., & Ling, W. (2003). The Clinical Opiate Withdrawal Scale (COWS). *J Psychoactive Drugs*, 35(2), 253–9.

Figure 6.3 COWS scale for opioid withdrawal symptoms

There are essentially 3 medications (FDA approved) for opioid maintenance or MAT:

Buprenorphine (Subutex): buprenorphine is a long-acting "weak" opioid that keeps the opioid receptor happy (no cravings or withdrawal), while also not being strong enough to get a "high" from. There is now an injection form (Sublocade), taken one time a week as well. Common side effects include headache, constipation, nausea, low blood pressure, numbness or burning of the mouth, serious – breathing slows or stops, and serious – liver damage.

Methadone: the first and mainline treatment for opioid addiction. Often controversial due to the perception of its dependence and "having a hold on people," methadone is a long-acting opioid that is taken once per day, typically by a liquid, and works similarly to buprenorphine. The goal is to keep the opioid system happy and to not have any cravings or withdrawal. Common side effects include anxiety, nervousness, restlessness, insomnia, weakness, drowsiness, dry mouth, nausea/vomiting, constipation, low appetite, low sex drive or difficulty having an orgasm, serious – breathing slows or stops, serious – hallucinations, and serious – high heart rate.

Naltrexone (Revia): naltrexone is not an opioid. Naltrexone works by blocking opioids from working in the brain. When taking naltrexone, if the person takes any opioids (such as trying to abuse them), the naltrexone will block the effect. This can help retrain the brain that there is no use to use opioids for abuse and further deter further usage. Naltrexone comes in a once-a-month injection form (Vivitrol), along with an implanted pump option that can last six months. Common side effects include nausea/vomiting, decreased appetite, dizziness, depression, anxiety, and high dosages – liver damage.

*****Suboxone** is a combo drug of buprenorphine and naloxone (Narcan). While the buprenorphine makes the opioid site happy (no cravings or withdrawal symptoms), the naloxone will block any opioids that the person may take to get a "high" from.

MAT doesn't have to be forever. There are some people who are on MAT for

5, maybe ten years, then decide that they are in a good place to try and taper off of MAT. One of the successful sides to MAT (although typically skipped over) is the use of psychotherapy, specifically cognitive behavioral therapy (CBT). The goal of treatment is to treat the addiction with a multifaceted approach. Having an addiction is traumatic and fearful; special self-care is needed no matter the treatment approach taken.

Methamphetamine and Stimulant Treatment

In the many years of addiction treatment, we haven't had much luck in creating a stimulant specific treatment. Stimulants continue to wreak havoc on families everywhere, and yet, the focus on the issue has been almost null. Stimulant addiction can be very difficult to treat, mostly because it is so readily available and cheap to use. One research article I was reading related good methamphetamine treatment to "drug testing" to keep accountability. Is this how far we have come? Some good news suggests that stimulant addiction can have some successful treatment from general addiction treatments already being used. Group counseling, individual therapy, and mental health can be just enough to help somebody out of stimulant addiction. Presently, there are no medications specifically made for the treatment of stimulants. One medication that is being studied is the medication naltrexone (Revia). Some preliminary studies show that naltrexone may ward off the feelings of high from stimulants, along with reducing the addictive, learned pattern. Naltrexone works by decreasing opioid response, but we have learned the opioid system in our body is closely functioning with the brain chemical dopamine which skyrockets with stimulant abuse. By indirectly blocking dopamine, stimulants may not get the person "high." This would make the person's motivation to try the stimulants again, much less.

Crack and Cocaine Treatment

While crack and cocaine are not as prominent as they used to be, people still suffer from addiction to either one. Like methamphetamine and stimulants, there are no specific treatments for crack and cocaine. Most treatments involve traditional addiction treatments, including group counseling, individual therapy, and treatment for any underlying mental health issues. Part of what ended the crack epidemic was that the prices rose so fast, along with being made with more impurities. There is also an unfortunate fact that much of the crack epidemic was overshadowed by the opioid epidemic, inadvertently hiding the crack users from the public spotlight.

Currently, there are no specific medications for crack or cocaine use.

12 step and SMART Recovery

One of the biggest impacts of addiction recovery has been that of the 12 step movement. Started by Bill Wilson and Dr. Robert Holbrook Smith in 1935 as Alcoholics Anonymous, 12 step has grown into one of the largest self-help groups in the world for addiction treatment. Since Alcoholics Anonymous, there have been splits into other areas, such as Narcotics Anonymous, Marijuana Anonymous, Overeaters Anonymous, and more. 12 step is based on 12 steps one must take to get rid of using any said substance.

The 12 Steps

1. We admitted we were powerless over our addiction, that our lives had become unmanageable.
2. Came to believe a Power greater than ourselves could restore us to sanity.

3. Made a decision to turn our will and our lives over to the care of God as we understand God.
4. Made a searching and fearless moral inventory of ourselves.
5. Admitted to God, to ourselves and to another human being the exact nature of our wrongs.
6. We're entirely ready to have God remove all these defects of character.
7. Humbly asked God to remove our shortcomings.
8. Made a list of all persons we had harmed and became willing to make amends to them all.
9. Made direct amends to such people wherever possible, except when to do so would injure them or others.
10. Continued to take personal inventory and when we were wrong, promptly admitted it.
11. Sought through prayer and meditation to improve our conscious contact with God as we understood God, praying only for the knowledge of God's will for us and the power to carry that out.
12. Having had a spiritual awakening as the result of these steps, we tried to carry this message to other addicts, and to practice these principles in all our affairs.

As most can tell, 12 step has a "higher power" component. Traditionally, this has meant a God, but many people in 12 step will inform you that 12 step is not a religious organization, nor do you have to have the higher power be a certain God. It simply means "a higher power that you understand to be higher and more powerful than you." Still, the idea of submitting to a "higher power" to some can be very uncomforting, especially those who don't believe in any sort of deity. 12 step also tends to view addiction as a moralistic issue. This can be conflicting to the 12 step belief that addiction is also a brain disease. I'm not sure that we could tell someone with a brain disease, like dementia, that they are immoral for their behaviors from dementia.

Another important aspect of 12 step is that not every group is the same. It is well known in the 12 step community which groups you can go to and score drugs. It's also known which ones you can go to and complete the "13th step" or getting romantically involved with another 12 step member. 12 step has also been for years, very reluctant to have any official research done on its effectiveness. It's for this reason that professionals in the mental health community recommend 12 step as an adjunctive therapy; that is, a therapy that is also a part of an evidenced-based therapy, such as cognitive behavioral therapy (CBT). This is not to say that literally millions of people who had addictions found solace and relinquishment from addiction through 12 step. I have seen many people who have successfully stopped their addiction through the use of 12 step. Being in a community of people who suffer the same as you is incredibly empowering, let alone, feeling able to help yourself by seeing examples in real-time. 12 step is also advantageous because of its availability in many cities, along with being free for all members. Truly, the access to the 12 step demonstrates how pathetic the rest of healthcare is to access of care to people with addiction.

SMART Recovery (Smart Management And Recovery Training) is another free, community setting addiction treatment. SMART recovery can be an alternative to those who have difficulty with a 12 step approach. SMART recovery has a non-higher power approach and generally views the "powerless" aspect of 12 steps to be detrimental to motivation. SMART recovery also sees addiction as a temporal state, rather than a permanent state as seen in the 12 step. I've talked to many people in 12 step who will tell me they are an "addict," and then when I ask what they are using, they state, "well, I drank alcohol 30 years ago and then stopped." SMART recovery would view this as not an addiction anymore as the behaviors have been extinguished. Is the person at risk for becoming addicted again? Sure. The same can be said of any medical condition. If you had cancer and then it was in remission, you wouldn't tell people you have cancer currently. You would state you "had" cancer. Now, cancer can reappear at any time at which, if it did, you would then go back to "having cancer." Also, SMART recovery's approach does not have you stand up and state, "Hello, my name is so and so, and I am an addict." Not that there's anything wrong with this approach by 12 step, but in SMART recovery, you are not required to tell what you are having difficulty controlling. I've seen people in SMART recovery for everything from heroin to nail-biting. SMART recovery's focus is on evidenced-based treatment, which includes cognitive behavioral skills along with distress tolerance skills. This approach can be appealing to people who are desiring something different than the 12 step approach. This is not to say that SMART recovery is better than 12 step, or vice versa. There are different approaches to community treatment, and finding what works (and doesn't work) for you is crucial to any success in battling addiction.

Need to connect to society

There is something to be said about our natural tendency to connect and be social with others. It is ingrained in our DNA to be social creatures. Addiction tends to rob people of socialization because addiction is such an isolating phenomenon. This isolation can take place either because family and loved ones have distanced themselves from you or because you have distanced yourself from them. For those who have been abused and traumatized, substances can provide more reliability and solace than humans. Many substances tap into oxytocin, the "bonding" brain chemical that allows us to connect with other humans. Not to mention dopamine, which then makes everyday interactions with others painfully boring, if not anxiety-ridden.

The more we research isolation in addiction, the more we understand how incredibly important it is to reconnect with humans in order to stave off addiction. Many times, a person's proneness to use substances is due to early childhood abuse. Gabor Maté, a Canadian psychiatrist in addiction in the downtown Vancouver heroin district, suggests that mistrust of people leads to distancing from them, but that craving for attachment is then met by substances. In my own practice, most people I see who have an addiction have some extensive trauma in their background, especially those who use multiple substances at the same time. This hasn't been helped much by our current, technological society. Think about it. You can walk about New York City today, with 8 million people in that city, and not say one word or interact with one person. This is not how humans were made to be. We flourish with cooperative interactions with others. We regulate our emotions and moods through humans. Addiction simply robs a person of that. So, when someone is seeking treatment for addiction, it's important for them to communicate and form new relationships with others. This may be how groups like 12 step work so well. The forming of a community can be very impactful to addiction treatment. Of course, there is a community for those who are addicted, but it tends to be a world where people are codependent, and the word "betrayal" is a common theme. This furthers a person into addiction as it reinforces the idea that humans are not to be trusted and certainly are a cause of harm. Healthy relationships with humans of healthy habits is a surer way to success from addiction anyways.

> To read more updates on addiction treatment, go to
> *virtuesofmentalhealth.com/addiction-medications*

12

UNIQUE POPULATIONS AND CONSIDERATIONS

"Always remember that you are absolutely unique. Just like everyone else."
-Margaret Mead

Older Adults

We have an increasingly aging population due to the baby boomers of the late 1940s and 1950s. By 2030, the US will have 1 in 5 people over the age of 65. All this occurring while childbirths are steadily lowering. Geriatrics (older adults) are a very important population with mental health needs. The shift from being a producer to maintaining health, loss of physical agility, and mental acuity play a significant role in the mental well-being of the aging person. Loss of friends, family, and others around an aging person may also affect their mental well-being. There are specific life events and transitions that occur when someone moves into older adulthood. Typically, legacy (what have I done with my life?) becomes the main focus.

Being human strivers, we can become depressed or upset if we feel we haven't achieved our goals or have done things that are regrettable. Because of this natural transition, there is a belief that depression is a normal part of aging. This is far from true. Depression is not a normal phenomenon in aging, just like anxiety is not a normal part of aging. If depression and anxiety are impairing the person's wellbeing and their ability to function in everyday life, then seeking treatment is necessary. Depression may be more common in older populations, though, and some studies show upwards of 15% of people over 65 have clinical depression (versus 7% of the general population). This can be very profound after the loss of a loved one or being diagnosed with a major illness. A topic we don't like to discuss but need to is suicide. Older populations generally are considered the highest risk of suicide (over 65). If you are white, male, and over age 55, you are five times more likely to actually attempt and complete suicide. Asking about suicidal thoughts is a must. There are no studies that show that asking about suicide makes people more suicidal. Generally, older populations present with a type of depression that gives low energy, poor concentration, and even memory issues. This can make it tough when trying to distinguish between depression and dementia. Eating, sleeping, and physical complaints are also very common in older populations with depression.

Memory loss isn't necessarily normal except in very mild cases. Dementia is an increasingly more common condition seen in older populations. Around 7% of people over age 60 have a form of dementia, and this number jumps dramatically when a person is 80 years or older (25-50%). Dementia generally falls into the realm of neurology, but dementia is very well known for having its mental health disturbances. As dementia increases in severity, mental health can begin to deteriorate rapidly. Impulsivity becomes an issue, maybe rage, or even violence may be possibilities in people who otherwise would have never done these behaviors before. A surprising statistic is the number of people who have dementia induced hallucinations and delusions. Upwards of 75% of people with dementia have hallucinations and delusions. Generally, treatment for dementias are medications that help slow down the progression of the disease. Psychiatric medications can be used to help control agitation or dangerous behaviors, along with hallucinations and delusions. Unfortunately, all dementias consume the functioning brain, and families take a big toll on deciding the care and treatment of their loved one. It truly is a devastating disease and we, as a nation, need to put our research and funding efforts towards a possible cure or better management.

Anxiety in aging populations tends to focus on physical issues. It can be difficult to determine if anxiety in older populations is from a mental health disturbance or a medical condition. Chronic illnesses, like thyroid issues, diabetes, heart issues, brain diseases, and more, can mimic or induce anxiety in older populations. Interestingly, generalized anxiety disorder (GAD) and obsessive-compulsive disorder (OCD) are the more common anxiety in the older population. OCD presents differently than in other age groups, as older populations tend to have OCD symptoms more related to handwashing and "feelings of dirtiness" or "having sinned" compared to typical OCD symptoms that can include issues with symmetry, counting, and rituals, such as flipping on the lights three times, etc. Often, worry and nervousness are the common factors in older populations with anxiety. While some anxiety can be normal in older populations, the level of impairment from the anxiety is the key to focus on. If they are being robbed of quality of life, then treatment ought to be sought.

Is it medical or psychological?

In younger populations, mental health symptoms can generally be assumed to be mental health issues (although not always!). Older populations face an array of medical ailments that can create mental health symptoms. For instance, a urinary tract infection is no fun for the person experiencing it, but older people can get delirious, even confused from the urinary tract infection. Other examples could be related to electrolyte imbalance or dehydration, which are more frequent in older populations. Hormones begin to shift, the brain begins to age more, and the body's ability to regulate because harder and harder. Tough to hear, but we will all go through these stages. Mental symptoms can be seen as the body's alarm system going off, telling you that something in the body is not working correctly, so it's always important to be seen by a primary care doctor along with any referred specialists (including a psychiatrist).

Here are some things to look out for that may indicate an underlying medical condition:

1. Is it a very sudden onset, or did it rapidly just appear? Generally speaking, mental illnesses creep in overtime rather than having a rapid onset
2. Is there a history of mental illness? Conditions like bipolar and schizophrenia almost always start earlier in a person's life. Ages 17 - 30 are typically years these conditions will start to show
3. Was there a new medication or treatment just started? All medications have some side effects, and our bodies are unique in how it handles them. Side effects from certain medication can cause mental symptom
4. Is the person seeing many doctors and being prescribed many medications? Polypharmacy (or taking many different medications at once) is a common phenomenon in the United States and medications can interact with each other, which can cause mental symptoms

Psychiatric Medication Considerations and Older Adults

When considering medications for older populations, you want to look at how the body will handle the medication. What does this mean? This means seeing if the kidneys are working properly, the liver, the digestive system, the heart, and the brain. These are all important organs that are responsible for how the medication will work. If anyone's system is not functioning properly, the special considerations need to be taken in the choice of medication and dosing of the chosen medication. I worked with a psychiatrist at a hospital at the beginning of my nursing journey who once told me that it's easy to figure out the dosage for older populations, "simply look for the starting dose normally used and cut it in half." If it were only that easy, many more considerations need to be taken to care for people.

*side note: this psychiatrist also didn't believe that borderline personality disorder was "real" and resigned from the hospital after being found urinating in the elevators

Psychotherapy Considerations and Older Adults

Life is hard, for everyone, some more than others. Transitioning to an older age is always a hard pill to swallow. Lost independence, ability to complete tasks, legacy issues are all very real concerns. Therapy can be very beneficial to help cope with this life transition. I find that most effective therapies for older populations involve finding meaning and positive regard for their life. While therapies like CBT and psychodynamic therapy are very good therapies, it can be challenging with older populations because their ways of thinking and coping have been hardwired for many years. This is not to say we shouldn't try these therapies, but be open to a different angle of approach to therapy. Specialized therapies, such as narrative therapy and acceptance and commitment therapy (ACT), along with interpersonal therapy, have very good evidence for their effect in older populations with mental illness or difficulties in transition.

Children and Adolescents

Children are not little adults. They have specific needs that need different approaches when compared to adults. Child mental health continues to be a big and diverse field, yet, the field is generally gutted financially and with very little clinician resources available. Historically, child mental health was not a major focus in the mental health community. Prior to the 20th century, children were viewed as having little to no worries, and any abnormal behaviors were either punished by the caregivers, handled by the legal system, or handled by the church. The first mental treatment for children was deemed to be "juvenile delinquency" centers, entailing that these youth with mental illness were deviant and disobedient. It wasn't until 1946 that Harry Truman signed the National Mental Health Act and the initiation of The American Association of Child Psychiatry in 1953 that child mental health became a serious topic of interest. Child-specific illnesses and comprehensive child treatment became a major research focus during the 1970s and 1980s.

Even with such advancements in child mental health, we still face grave disparities in the specialized field of children and adolescents. Some of the ills are simply the lack of inpatient hospital beds for children with mental illnesses. It didn't necessarily use to be this way. With high liability and reports of high seclusion and restraint use, many child inpatient units began to shut down or convert to adult-only units. Inpatient mental health already has difficulty obtaining payment for the cost of treatment, the lawsuits, and mental health rights advancing in child mental health was the last nail in the coffin. We certainly did need to address, and yes, shut down the deplorable conditions in some of the child inpatient units, but we face a massive shortage of inpatient child mental health beds, making a severely mentally ill child, who may want to hurt themselves or others, left to try and be managed in an outpatient setting. Another critical issue in child mental health is the use of psychiatric medications. There is no doubt that some children will desperately need psychiatric medication(s), but how we determine this and how safely we can manage psychiatric medications in children can become challenging. Many of the psychiatric medications we use in children are not FDA approved to be used in children. That doesn't mean this is malpractice or not appropriate. It simply means that the FDA has looked at all the extensive clinical trials of the medication on adults only. Most psychiatric medications for children are dosed and considered safe based on adult studies of the medication. This can be problematic as children are not the same as adults as far as their metabolism or how their body will react with the medications. Most are very safe and used without issue, but we do need to focus on getting more studies on psychiatric medications for children, especially on long term use during development. Why has there been no studies with children?

Liability is the simplest answer. Most parents are also not willing to have their child be used in research due to potential adverse reactions, and this is very understandable. So, this makes child mental health challenging from a psychiatric medication perspective. To partly remedy this, child psychiatry is much more reluctant to give psychiatric medications to a child and is more geared towards an approach that focuses on therapy and comprehensive team approaches. Children are also still developing, and their brains are very resilient and able to rebuild more effectively than adults. This makes therapy and team approach with many mental health disciplines much more advantageous as it helps to rebuild the child's brain and helps with their natural development. Psychiatric medications are important, especially if there is psychosis, severe depression, and bipolar disorder. It is always important to know that medications don't ever replace a good comprehensive treatment team; it is merely a sliver of the whole pie.

Children being different than adults leads to children having different mental conditions, or more prevalent mental health conditions. Some go into adulthood, others don't. Some are because of trauma and abuse, some are purely genetic or brain structure issues. Some are all of the above. Below is a short synapse of the common childhood mental health conditions. It should be noted that you may see overlap, and this is definitely not a full, exhaustive list of childhood mental health conditions. Always seek out professional help when determining what the most appropriate diagnosis is.

Oppositional Defiant Disorder (ODD) - Children with ODD are very often arguing with adults, losing their tempers, and can be very resentful and easily annoyed with others. Generally, these events are grossly out of proportion to the actual dialogue or requests of the adults. The focus of hostility and disobedience is almost always towards those of authority, which can include parents, teachers, law enforcement, and other figures. Actions can be simply not following through with requests to breaking the rules and purposely trying to agitate others. One important factor in ODD is that the child doesn't generally act with physical assault. If a physical assault occurs frequently, then conduct disorder may be a diagnosis to look at. To be diagnosed with ODD, these deviances have to occur over six months. Children with ODD often have an external locus of control, that is, they tend to feel that their actions are due to what others do to them and generally don't take any responsibility for them.

Conduct Disorder - Conduct disorder is more than just a "behavioral child." Conduct disorder is a child who frequently violates the basic rights of people, which can include violence, manipulation, stealing, and destruction of property. Lying can be a hallmark feature of conduct feature, along with a substantial lack of remorse or guilt. Children with conduct disorder are frequent visitors to the juvenile system. The signs of conduct disorder are not an "overnight" phenomena, but rather a gradual presentation of behaviors. Conduct disorder can be very treatment-resistant, meaning that it can be difficult to treat and effectively get results. Unfortunately, many children and adolescents with conduct disorder turn 18 and "graduate" to a diagnosis of antisocial personality disorder.

Disruptive Mood Dysregulation Disorder (DMDD) - severe tantrums and easily provoked, the child with DMDD is easily triggered to have explosive anger. In between these explosive episodes, the child is generally very negative, irritable, or sad most of the time. This disorder is more commonly seen in males than in females. It also overlaps quite a bit with other impulse disorders, such as ODD, conduct disorder, bipolar disorder, and ADHD.

Separation Anxiety - most children feel comforted with their caregiver(s) and feel some anxiety when that person is not around, but children with separation anxiety are a step beyond this. Intense dread, panic, and worry are classic features of separation anxiety. Generally, there may be a precipitating event, such as moving to a new home, death of a family member or friend, or serious injury event. In these cases, you may see the child begin to fear that something will happen to the caregiver if they are to separate. Refusal to go to school, play with friends, to spend the night somewhere may be commonplace in separation anxiety. At times, an emotionally overbearing parent may put pressure (inadvertently) on the child, who then feels responsible for the parent's care. It may even be that the child is scared that this parent will die without them there to "help" them. The majority of cases generally dissipate, sometimes to complete opposites, where the child begins to rebel and speak coldly of the caregiver. Generally, children with separation anxiety have a parent with a moderate to severe anxiety disorder. Therapy is generally the best approach to separation anxiety.

Disinhibited Social Engagement Disorder & Reactive Attachment Disorder - often seen in children who have been abused or neglected, we have two types of attachment styles that may arise. Disinhibited social engagement disorder is a loose attachment style; generally, on the edge of promiscuous, they will be incredibly outgoing and boldly clinging to strangers. This may be met with complete indifference to their actual caregivers and appear to have altered their secure attachment to another figure within minutes. Reactive attachment, on the other hand, is the complete opposite of disinhibited social engagement disorder. Reactive attachment disorder presents with children who do not have any desire to attach to any caregiver. Children with reactive attachment have origins related to trauma (abuse or neglect). Reactive attachment can be so severe that a child may become a "failure to thrive" state. This is where the child fails to eat, and bodily functions begin to fail. Both disinhibited social engagement disorder and reactive attachment disorder are generally treated with nourishing relationships with caregivers who are trained to help the child rebuild secure attachments.

Child-Specific Wisdom Points

Children tend to present with mental conditions differently than adults, throwing caregivers off guard when they learn that their child is having mental health issues. Getting children to actually engage in treatment is another obstacle often faced by caregivers who are trying to help their child. Most children, like adults, crave to be perceived as "normal" and to be accepted amongst their peers. Social pressure is incredibly strong during childhood and adolescent years, not to mention that children can be incredibly resilient, even in the worst of situations. I hear so much from adults who were hurting so much as a child state that nobody had a clue as to their hurt. The desire to be lovable and accepted means that a lot of children end up sacrificing everything about themselves in order to please their caregivers, family, and friends. Children are highly loyal beings. Their desire to be loyal to caregivers and to be loved by them can create confusion for many caregivers who feel that their child is doing "just fine." This is no fault to most caregivers, who are typically caught blind sighted when they learn of their child's suffering. It's always important to always have "mental checks" with your kids to explore their reality and to create a "safe space" where they can explain their feelings and thoughts without any consequences.

Stated again, children express mental conditions differently than adults. Some good tips for identifying if your child or adolescent has any mental conditions is the following:

Depression: Children who are depressed tend to express depression as irritability and anger. Children also tend to express depression as "body pains," or physical manifestations like stomach aches, headaches, fatigue, and others. Depressed children tend to have lower energy than other children in the same age group. Their desire to play with other friends and children is generally distanced and withdrawn. This isolating behavior can be a safeguard to protect their hurting from children who may make fun of their apparent differences in interaction from other children.

Anxiety: Anxiety in childhood is one of the most common types of mental issues. It can be very hard to determine what is an anxiety problem versus normal anxiety in childhood. We certainly expect a child to be anxious when a parent is away, or when they face the first day at a new school. When a child is refusing to go to school because they fear their caregiver will die, we might have reached a level that is considered necessary for treatment. These children who fear to go to school may have anxiety related to a caregiver dying, but also to failing or being rejected by peers. Children with anxiety, like depression, tend to express their anxiety in the form of physical complaints. "Tummy aches" and "headaches" tend to be the most common forms of complaints. Frequent visits to the nurse's station at school can also be a sign of high anxiety. Bullying is a sad, but common occurrence. We may need to further investigate any childhood anxiety due to bullying at school. Whatever the cause it, the general pattern in children with anxiety tends to be an avoidance pattern; that is, they will avoid the cause of the anxiety. The expression of physical complaints is mostly due to their inability to express what "anxiety" is.

Abuse: Child abuse is more common than we can ever believe. Children who are being abused respond in many ways that often confuse the caregivers. Around one-third of children who experience a traumatic event are able to be resilient to any symptoms from it, which can last into adulthood. Most, though, face heavy mental tribulations following any type of traumatic and abusive event(s). Children who are abused tend to show expressions of the "extremes," meaning that they tend to be extreme in one way or the complete opposite way. For instance, when a child is sexually abused, they may express this abuse as either being overtly sexual for their age level, or they may be so passive on sexual topics that they appear to be almost to the level of a nun. This "nun" factor may include statements of absolute disgust in regard to any sexual topic, or statements of being "dirty" or something wrong with their private areas. One major red flag in sexual abuse is when the child becomes infatuated with sexual topics and begins to express sexual interest in others. This can be expressed by statements, behaviors, and informs of drawings/art or internet searches. Anger, agitation, tantrums, and violent behaviours may also be indicative of abuse occurring. Frequent school disruptions and general despise towards adults can be a red flag. Any sudden shift in connection to a family member or certain adult may also indicate a possible abuse that has occurred between that adult and child, or that the child is reminded of an abuser by that certain adult. One of the biggest red flags is when a child begins to hurt animals or other children. Children who severely abuse or kill animals merely express their desire to attempt to gain the control that was taken away from them by the same act that made them feel out of control. If you feel absolutely out control by a certain act, the mind will think that you need to do that act in order to gain control. It should also be noted that children who are harming or killing animals may be indicative of conduct disorder, a precursor to antisocial personality disorder.

Seeking help for any childhood mental conditions can be very challenging. There is a national shortage of child mental health professionals, especially in the psychiatric field. Adequate mental health counseling in schools is often gutted, and many children are missed in the system that needs help then and there. When seeking treatment, I am a big advocate in seeking psychotherapy before the introduction of medications. With a few exceptions like schizophrenia, bipolar, and ADHD, medications can merely mask an issue that is occurring in the child's environment. Children's brains are very resilient, and if there is a time to learn adaptive coping and new ways of thinking, childhood is the best time to do so. Only after therapy and with a recommendation from mental health professionals, would I consider giving a child psychiatric medication.

Whatever the case is, when it comes to children, it is always to be safe than sorry. Seeking treatment for a child can be a difficult decision, but the rewards to be reaped can be very beneficial to the child's future. So many of my patients' tribulations start in childhood, only to be exacerbated by lack of understanding and further delving into deeper trouble. There is no shame in bringing the opportunity for a child to be well again.

For more about child abuse, go to Chapter 13 "The Trauma Manifesto"

Military

The United States military continues to be one of the more prominent topics in mental health, and for a good reason. Wars and combat are nothing more than every human's worst nightmare. There's more than just the risk of being killed or having a fellow soldier killed or maimed. Military training involves making the average human into a trained killing machine. This certainly has a number of effects in the human psyche, which is generally averse to harming other humans. Trauma and PTSD are one of my passions in treatment. I tend to gravitate towards people who suffer from horrendous acts by humans or disasters. Yet, my knowledge and experience with the military culture lacked in many ways. I was lucky to be able to practice at the PTSD clinic at the VA in Long Beach, California, where my eyes were truly opened to a completely new realm of mental health issues in the military.

Military Culture and Mindset

Any person who is in the military knows the first and foremost goal is to protect the country. As we continue to have wars and fight other humans, the military is trained to do so. Although the majority of the military will not see any combat, the training alone creates mindsets that are attuned to combat, but not for everyday civilian living. Training in the military, first and foremost, makes a distinction between "us and them". This type of thinking makes it easy for people in the military to be able to draw distinct lines between what is "right" and what is "wrong". In addition to this, what is "wrong" needs to be neutralized. This could mean the person stating that it's "wrong" or by the extreme of actually killing the "wrong". This can be troublesome in civilian life because the military mindset can be very black and white; that is "it's this way or that way." This rigidity makes it very difficult for people who are trained by the military to live in a civilian world that is diverse and complex. The military loves simple answers, it makes decisions much easier. In many ways, the military is like our base humanity. As humans, we like simple answers as well as it makes it easier to make things more predictable. Imagine being a part of a system that completely reinforces that? We are already prone to black and white thinking and all or nothing, along with me versus them.

This rigidity that is trained in the military culture is continued into the civilian world. Rigid ideas of the world lead to some irritability to outright rage and violence towards others. When there is rigidity in thought, there is a strong "right vs. wrong," which plays into every situation. The "I am right; you are wrong" mentality isn't unique to the military but is more common. This wreaks havoc on relationships and parental involvement. This, sadly, can be a contributing factor to the very high military divorce rates seen. When there is a tendency to "squash" any "threat," there can be many possible scenarios that make it difficult to work with others, let alone form long-lasting and deep relationships that are bound to have differences of opinion. This is not to say that people in the military are bad people. Quite the contrary, their service leads to sacrifices that are seen by these events in their relationships. We talk about combat, deaths, and injuries as sacrifices, but the unspoken of sacrifice that may be more so is the sacrifice that they have on their mental health and their relationships with others.

Military PTSD

PTSD is well known in the military, although most people in the United States don't get PTSD from the military. That honor goes to car accidents. But the interest and research into PTSD always come in times of war when we see soldiers who start to develop debilitating PTSD. While PTSD in the military has a lot of similar features to any other type of PTSD, PTSD in the military also can present very differently. PTSD in the military tends to be an exaggeration of the training they received, at least in civilian life. Aspects of PTSD are very helpful in a combat zone. Being hypervigilant, precautious of others, and easily startled can save your life or that of your unit. In civilian life, this can be viewed as paranoia, anger, and inability to connect with others. Indeed, military people with PTSD are typically presented with more of these types of PTSD symptoms (hypervigilance, agitation, and inability to trust others). The disconnect from military life to civilian has also shown the propensity to have PTSD symptoms. When you are in a combat zone, these PTSD symptoms are accepted and honed into the combat. In civilian life, they are drastically different than the average civilian's way of dealing with stress. This makes it painfully obvious to the soldier, who then feels out of place in a world that they sacrificed to keep as it. Many veterans with PTSD have a core issue with feeling safe. "Perimeter checks" at night around their house may keep them up all night. Traffic on the highway may make them feel completely out of control because they feel that they don't have an escape route to be safe. Being in any situation where you feel stuck makes you feel incredibly vulnerable and at a high risk of being killed. In a civilian world that doesn't understand this, the alienation and isolation that is seen with many people who were in the military begin to fester.

A high "threat detection" alarm in PTSD can make living day to day incredible painful and extraneous. I remember treating a Vietnam Vet who had ongoing PTSD since 1978. He was a bus driver. When a patron would challenge him on paying for the bus ride, he would blackout and the next thing he remembered was the guy on the ground outside the bus with a bloody nose. Another Vietnam Vet I treated was banned from the strawberry stand, where they bought fresh strawberries every season because he punched the owner of the stand for "allowing another patron to cut" in front of him. It's no surprise that these knee jerk reactions and locking horns with others can lead many veterans with PTSD in a lot of trouble. Extreme and risky behaviors may also be a factor. High speeding on a motorcycle, crazy attempts at tricks on a dirt bike, racing cars, fighting, and any other extreme sport can be common in veterans. The thrills and high energy activities that are seen in combat make a veteran incredibly bored with normalcy in civilian life. This addiction to adrenaline that they feel makes them want to do activities that match the extreme nature of their mind. Doing extreme behaviors also gives a false illusion that they are in control when they feel out of control most of the time. Imagine traveling 115 MPH on a motorcycle in traffic. Very dangerous and high risk, coupled with lots of anxiety. If the person makes it to their destination without any harm, this gives the false illusion that they were in control of high a risk and dangerous situation. This can be incredibly relieving to the constant feeling that they are out of control in the majority of their life. Couple this with flashbacks, where they feel that they are right back in combat or nightmares that frequent weekly and you have a person who is constantly being dragged back to the combat they faced and robbing them of the present moment that they sacrificed to keep the same.

Military and Treatment

If there is a mental health condition that is deemed to be attributed to their military time, it is always worth it to see if they can get service connected to a VA healthcare facility. The VA, not perfect by any means, has some of the best evidence and researched backed treatments for military veterans. This treatment is literally world-renowned and is not only free to veterans with service-connection, but sometimes the veteran can receive a monetary benefit from the service-connected illness. When the VA is not an option, say in a dishonorable discharge, then seeking out civilian treatment is necessary. When seeking out treatment for military PTSD, you want to find a therapist who specializes in trauma treatments, such as cognitive processing therapy, prolonged exposure therapy, or eye movement desensitization reprocessing. The medication treatment for military PTSD is relatively the same as PTSD treatment for any other trauma-related event. Couples therapy may also be necessary as relationships suffer heavily from military PTSD. More and more, the military is seeking out ways to prevent PTSD in their service members, but it is an uphill fight as the nature of the military is to be trained to combat other humans, and that will always make it a high risk for PTSD and other related mental conditions. Even with re-integration advancements by the military to put soldiers back into civilian life, we still see a high prevalence of soldiers, especially those in combat, having PTSD symptoms.

Lesbian, Gay, Bisexual, Trans, and Queer (LGBTQ)

To see how far we have come in the past 20 years in LGBTQ acceptance and legislation is truly astonishing. From homosexuality being the most "sinful" of forms of love to a nation where same-sex marriage is legal and more readily accepted is truly something to experience and shows that we are able, as humans, to advance our ability to accept others and incorporate new ways of learning. This should be a positive to see in our human species. Yet, people in the LGBTQ community continue to face stigma and bullying that is detrimental to their mental health. When you are a part of the 4.5 - 5% of U.S. adults who identify with the LGBTQ community, you face the psychological tribulations that are faced by being a minority. When coming of age and beginning to find your sexuality, we all find ourselves in an awkward space. Sex and attraction are already uncomfortable topics to discuss as a coming to age child, let alone when you have feelings that differ from what you heard is "normal." This confusion that most feel causes extreme anxiety, depression, and feelings of "defectiveness." Imagine it, you are lined up in a group of 20 people, and you are the only one who is completely different than the other 19 in terms of sexuality. That's incredibly scary and isolating. As creatures who want to fit in and be loved, people in the LGBTQ community tend to beat themselves up over their apparent "difference" from others. To face such adversity so early in life makes all the sense why people in the LGBTQ community face higher numbers of mental health conditions.

Sexuality is an incredibly complex development, and the idea of "normal" development sexuality is generally challenged by any observation of people. Think of all the different ways people express their sexuality. To put a manual on how to be sexual would be the worst publications ever produced. What we all tend to agree on are healthy relationships where there is a connection and no harm.

One of the factors in mental health in the LGBTQ community is the stigma that can arise within the community. You may find some gay men who despise drag queens or gay men who despise trans people. You may see trans people who separate themselves greatly from lesbians and gays as they feel that they are a separate group from them. In any sense, the public tends to see the LGBTQ as a cohesive group, but this is further from the truth. This splintering also creates division and further alienation from feeling a part of other humans. People who are trans or "other" feel the most stigma as even those who are gay and lesbian fight to be a part of the "norm." This isn't to say that all gays, lesbians, bisexuals, trans, and queer hate each other. Just go to pride parade, and you'll see all these communities come together for a common cause. This is a common phenomenon that is seen in any minority. Blacks may discriminate against "whiter" or "lighter" skinned blacks, and vice versa. Lighter skinned Asian populations may view darker-skinned Asians as lesser than thou. So, this isn't unique to the LGBTQ community but contributes to some of the higher prevalence in mental health conditions.

Seeking treatment in the LGBTQ community should be sought by a professional who is familiar with the LGBTQ community issues. In the end, it's important to remember that our struggles to be human and thrive in this world are not just unique to my "normality," but to any human who is born on this earth.

13

A TRAUMA MANIFESTO

"There are wounds that never show on the body that are deeper and more hurtful than anything that bleeds."
-Laurell K. Hamilton

Many people hear of psychological trauma and posttraumatic stress disorder (PTSD) from news coverage of a serial killer's torturous sprees, or combat soldiers in wars in countries far away. This isn't by coincidence. Historically, trauma and PTSD are generally put in the spotlight during wars. "Shell shock" during World War One, "War Neurosis" in World War Two, and finally PTSD in the Vietnam War. These type of traumatic symptoms were considered a cost of war, although, during World War One, some soldiers with shell shock were executed for what was thought to be desertion. The only other time "trauma" was a research topic with any widespread interest was the study of "hysteria" in the late 19th century. Hysteria comes from the Latin word, *hystera*, or uterus. This isn't by mistake as hysteria was believed to be a "women's" condition. Jean-Martin Charcot tried adamantly to dispel that females were only prone to "hysteria" by bringing in some male patients who displayed "hysteria," but his attempt at changing the tides of 19th-century European views on women couldn't stick.

Sigmund Freud studied hysteria extensively and was one of the first in history to attribute it to past trauma, along with Pierre Janet and Jean-Martin Charcot in France. At the time, Freud was seeing patients with hysteria in the academic setting in Vienna. Most of these women were prostitutes, homeless, or in abject poverty. For Freud, the hysterics seen were a result of trauma that occurs at "this level" of society. His writings and research on what we would call PTSD today was truly astonishing and was years ahead of its time. Unfortunately, and tragically, Freud began working with high aristocratic families to earn more money as the academic setting was not lucrative. When Freud discovered that hysteria was occurring in women in his same social class and acts like incest, sexual abuse, and neglect were also occurring, he simply could not handle that his social class did these things. In many ways, this is when we see Freud shift from trauma-based hysteria to more sexually based conflicts that we have come to know with Freudian theory. This didn't help females by any means who were already stigmatized as "emotionally vulnerable" to hysteria. Now they were to have a component that demonstrated their deep sexual conflicts, further stigmatizing women as inferior to morals and emotional stoicism that "males" had. It wouldn't be till the late 20th century that research studying trauma and PTSD saw the genius that Freud demonstrated in those early papers. It's unfortunate there were almost hidden from sight; I wonder how much further we would be in trauma treatments having used the research much earlier.

PTSD wasn't a diagnosis until 1980 when it was included in the DSM texts. Of course, we know that trauma is nothing new. Humanity and the animal kingdom can be incredibly cruel. The systems involved in trauma and PTSD are there to protect us. But when this system is hit hard or activated over and over, our mental health deteriorates even more than we could ever believe. In the mental health field, we always had an idea that abuse and adverse events, especially in childhood, could lead to mental health issues. It seems completely obvious and sensible. What we failed to understand for many decades was the true impact of trauma not just on mental health, but physical health, and even the life span. The true impact of trauma was unexpectedly discovered with a study that, inadvertently, had nothing to do with trauma and mental health per se. It was a big study on obesity, but what came from this one study opened the floodgates and changed the face of mental health forever.

Adverse Childhood Experiences (ACE) Study

It's 1995, and Dr. Felitti and Dr. Anda were trying to figure out what contributes to the growing obesity epidemic. Based out of the Kaiser Permanente Hospital System in San Diego, Dr. Felitti and Dr. Anda sought to gather an estimated 17,000 Kaiser members who were suffering from obesity. The idea? To see how their childhoods were. They were wondering if someone's childhood affected their eating behaviors later in life and if this was a contributing factor. To assess the participants, they created the Adverse Childhood Experiences scale or ACE. The ACE scale is 10 questions, with each "yes" being 1 point, equally a total of 10 points.

This ACE scale was given to the participants and was scored by the research team. What was found was truly astonishing and disturbing. 1 in 5 participants had a family member with mental illness. This isn't compelling as 1 in 5 U.S. adults have a diagnosable mental illness. 1 in 5 grew up in a dysfunctional household. More shocking, 1 in 5 were sexually abused as children, and 1 in 4 were physically abused as children. These numbers were disturbing. How is it that sexual and physical abuse are this common? It was truly the unraveling of a much-held secret in history. From this one study, came more studies about the ACE score and other risks of other ailments. Further studies showed that if you have an ACE score of 4 or more, you were 7x more likely to be an alcoholic, 30x more likely to attempt suicide, 2x more likely to get cancer, and 4x more likely to get emphysema. A score of 4 or more in children found that they are 32x more likely to have "behavioral" problems in school. 66% of women in the United States experienced family dysfunction, abuse, or violence.

Adverse Childhood Events (ACE) Scale
Before being 18 years old, did the following happen:
1. Did a parent or other adult in the household often or very often Swear at you, insult you, put you down, or humiliate you? Or Act in a way that made you afraid that you might be physically hurt?
2. Did a parent or other adult in the household often or very oftenPush, grab, slap, or throw something at you? or Ever hit you so hard that you had marks or were injured
3. Did an adult or person at least five years older than you ever Touch or fondle you or have you sexually touch their body? Or Attempt or have oral, anal, or vaginal intercourse with you?
4. Did you often or very often feel that No one in your family loved you or thought you were important or special? Or Your family didn't look out for each other, feel close to each other, or support each other?
5. Did you often or very often feel that You didn't have enough to eat, had to wear dirty clothes, and had no one to protect you? Or Your parents were too drunk or high to take care of you or take you to the doctor if you needed it?
6. Were your parents ever separated or divorced?
7. Was your mother or stepmother? Often or very often pushed, grabbed, slapped, or had something thrown at her? Or Sometimes, often, or very often kicked, bitten, hit with a fist, or hit with something hard? Or Ever repeatedly hit over at least a few minutes or threatened with a gun or knife?
8. Did you live with anyone who was a problem drinker or alcoholic, or who used street drugs?
9. Was a household member depressed or mentally ill, or did a household member attempt suicide?
10. Did a household member go to prison?
For every "yes" answer, that is 1 point. Add these "yes" answers and that is your ACE score

Table 8.1 ACE Questionnaire

The ACE score of 6 or more indicated that they are 46x more likely to use IV drugs. The ACE score of 4 or more was more 3x more likely to have more than 50 sexual partners. So, what did the ACE studies teach us? One, that abuse, and childhood strife is incredibly common, and two, that whenever a child experiences these events, it increases their risks substantially of having mental illness and chronic, physical diseases, and yes, possibly early death.

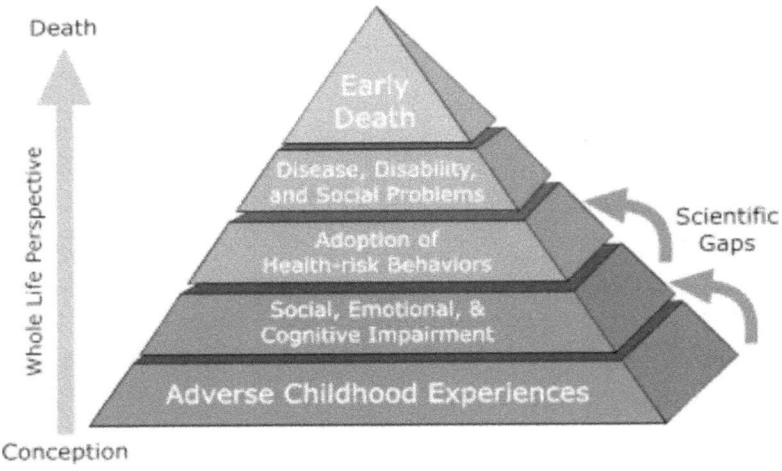

Figure 8.1 ACE Pyramid: ACE experiences lead to fundamental change

Child Abuse and Development

Children face abuse and trauma differently than adults and for obvious reasons. They are dependent on their caregivers, and the sphere of the world revolves around them. When a child is abused, either physically, emotionally, or sexually, they face great confusion about what adults do and how adults can be. This ultimately shapes their worldview in their developing years and, without intervention, will be solidified in adulthood. Sexual abuse, in particular, is incredibly damaging to a child's development. Shame, guilt, and secrecy are common themes experienced by children who are sexually abused. Such thoughts come from not understanding their role in a sexual context. Confusion about being a "willing participant" is also common and brings on shame. The "willing participant" thought may originate from the "pleasure" that they get from sexual abuse, or from their freezing behavior, which allows the abuse to occur without a struggle. One thing I counsel boys who may have been sexually abused is letting them know that if they got an erection during the abuse, that this doesn't mean they "liked it" or "wanted it," rather, it is a normal physical effect from stimulation. The "freezing" reaction stems from our prehistoric brain. Typically, when something threatening occurs, our brain puts us into "fight or flight" mode, making us want to fight the threat or try to escape. This may happen initially for most, but a person who is absolutely dominated and unable to escape will exhaust the "fight or flight" system and will go into a "freeze" and "dissociate" mode. Dissociating is your body's natural way to "escape" the horrendous act that is occurring. Dissociating is actually the dumping of your body's natural opioids (painkillers) into your bloodstream in order to numb you from the terrible experience. While your brain is trying to be nice to you, usually this will leave the child feeling confused because "they did nothing to stop it."

What can make this more challenging for any type of abuse is that children are naturally very loyal to adults and caregivers. Typically, the pressure internally to remain silent is high, thus leaving the child to try and comprehend the abuse in understandable ways. Remember when you were a child, and you got incredibly scared? What was the first thing you did? Ran to Mom? Dad? Our natural tendency is to attach more when we feel scared, and this attachment can even happen to the abuser, especially if the abuser is a caregiver neglecting the child. Extreme cases of this happens when a child that was abused by a parent or caregiver defends the abusive caregiver. Why does this happen? To a child, the parent who is not abusing the child may appear to be "allowing the abuse to occur," or showing indifference to it. The abuser, on the other hand, does abuse the child, but also "shows interest" in the child, even if it's negative. In a survival sense, it's more advantageous to attach to someone who shows interest in you and may be willing to take care of you than a person who may neglect and ignore you.

One phenomenon that occurs when a child is abused is that their sense of safety is completely shattered. Normal child development has a child experience life with their actions causing consequences. This teaches a child that they are individuals with their own choices and own self-control. This is crucial for later adulthood as a healthy and emotionally regulated adult who has a sense of self and an internal sense of control. An abused child gets robbed of this development milestone. To an abused child, being abused creates feelings of being out of control, dominated, and terrorized. Any sense of self-controlled safety and ability to control strong emotions is a complete no go. Instead, the child learns that they don't have control over very crucial things like safety, and emotional well-being. Instead, that has been taken and is now being done by an external force, the abuser. The phenomenon creates a child who develops with poor internal self-control. Instead, their perception is that everything is externally controlled, meaning that their safety is dependent on others and how they feel is also dependent on others. This leads to an adult life of being dependent on others for their feelings of safety and emotional well-being. Unfortunately, the only ones who are willing to connect to such dependent people may be abusive and dominating partners, thus completing the cycle of abuse from childhood to adulthood. This external feeling of control can also lead to the abused person feeling that they cannot do anything themselves. This is usually perceived by outsiders as a "lack of responsibility" or "blaming," when indeed, it is a result of being horribly traumatized.

How do abused people end up being with abusers again? In many ways, abuse and trauma lead a child down a different journey than your "average" child. Take a sexually abused girl. Her perception of the world is one that is with this sexual overtone. Important relationships are forever tainted with this component. Sexually abused girls are notoriously known to start puberty earlier than other girls. This is most likely due to the sexual abuse telling the body that they need to get ready quickly to be able to reproduce. When a girl goes through puberty early, or is emotionally having difficulties due to the abuse, other children notice. Children can be cruel, and their idea of anything "different" is typically met with disdain, bullying, or complete ignoring. Late childhood and teenage years are crucial for your ability to have friends that you can emotionally regulate with. Imagine, you experience jealousy, extreme thoughts in relationships like "we'll get married when I turn 18!" Or even thoughts of getting pregnant or fathering a baby. Your friends (for the most part) are the common sense group that helps you regulate these strong thoughts. Either by giving you advice or simply guilt-tripping you for thinking that way, a teenager learns why it's important to control and self-regulate emotions. Abused children may not get this opportunity if they are outcasted, leaving them to try and self-regulate themselves. If they aren't given those chances to experience strong emotions with subsequent chances to regulate them with friends, then they enter life with poorly regulated and very strong emotions.

Extreme begets extreme. How often have you heard a friend say, "hey, you should meet my friend, you guys would be cute together!" Only to have another friend say, "oh no, she's too wild and crazy, you wouldn't want to be with her!" While on the surface, this appears to be a "compatibility" mismatch, it also shows that people who are emotionally not regulated and "extreme" in their behaviors generally won't find a self-regulated or safe person. Instead, extreme will attract extreme, by choice, or merely little options. When you get a vulnerable and abused person whose reliance on the basics of safety and emotional connection is fragmented, you have invited the opportunity for someone who is controlling and willing to take the role completely and forcefully.

Abusive Relationships

Abusive relationships, sometimes called domestic violence or the newer, intimate partner violence, is another complicated trauma experienced by millions across the world. What makes abusive relationships complicated is the perceived "choice" that the people have in the relationship. Yes, these are adult relationships, and yes, technically, adults are more responsible and can make more choices than a child. But, the complications of relationships are incredible, and most people fail to recognize (or simply choose not to) the complexity that abusive relationships have, whether it's due to safety or high investment into the relationship. Rape is actually a common phenomenon in relationships, although this was never considered "rape" for much of human existence. We understand when a stranger gets raped that this is clearly and definitely wrong and bad. What makes things more complicated is if the person who was raped originally showed interest or even began a relationship with the person. Suddenly the waters get murkier, and it's very unfortunate because most of the time, the victim will be the one to be blamed or written off.

For more established relationships, an abused partner is merely seen as a "willing participant." How could anyone want to stay with someone who abuses them? Many people who end up as victims in abusive relationships know the pattern too well as they were probably abused before. Remember, abuse makes a person want to attach more, and generally to a "protector" or "dominating" figure. Factor in guilt, shame, low self-esteem, and the feelings of being "dirty" or "defective," and you have a person who is willing to attach to any figure who shows genuine interest, even if negative. Some liken abusive relationships to a slot machine. At first, you give just a little (25 cents) for what is potentially a big win. You keep investing a little bit more and more, and guess what? Sometimes you get a little reward for that investment, say some affection, or a gesture that is over the top romantic. You keep investing more and more, hoping for the "big change" or "big reward." Well, for most, if not all people, the house always wins. By the time you begin to wear out, you have invested so much into this machine that you will feel devastated to leave it behind. What was it for? What will people say? How could I get myself into this? Like the slot machine, to leave the relationship would be to leave a huge investment from your life, your energy, your love, and caring. This is what makes abusive relationships so resistant. To leave might also mean criticism from others you care about, "of course we knew it was wrong for you to be in that relationship" or "you should have known better" are comments all too common. There is enough guilt and shame in abusive relationships, the fear of taking on more of that is devastating.

It's also crucial to understand that leaving a violent partner is very dangerous. Abusers feed their self-worth and self-esteem by dominating and having control. Simply losing the ability to control someone can drive them to despair, which they handle with anger and violence. Upwards of 75% of murders in domestic violence couples is when the abused person tries to leave the abuser. Any attempt to leave is a sign to the abuser that they need to abuse faster and harder than before. Unfortunately, abused people know this all too well.

Trauma and Mental Illness

How much is trauma a part of mental illness? It's hard to grasp because of the complexity of mental illness and the brain. Genetics can be a very big factor. We are starting to learn though that genes can be altered by traumatic experiences, which are then passed onto offspring, making them more vulnerable to mental illnesses. There is no doubt that traumatic experiences can lead to mental health issues, but how much is the "cause" is still being investigated. There is a projection, though, and it's safe to say we learn about trauma the more we see how influential it is in the development of mental illnesses. The general population that has experienced at least one traumatic event in their life is upwards of 50 - 60%. On average, when a person walks into my office to see me, I can safely assume that 70 - 80% of them have experienced at least one traumatic event, and most of the time, more. One of the more troubling discoveries is the very high prevalence of auditory hallucinations with childhood sexual abuse. Trauma fundamentally alters the brain. The extreme strain put on the brain can lead to parts not being able to function well and do what they need to do. The brain is like a muscle; if we remember, what is "used more" becomes stronger, what is "not used," gets weaker. Thus, traumatic experiences train the brain's emotional center, especially the fear center. When emotions are strong, and there is fear, other parts of the brain that help us control those emotions are now weaker. When this happens, we have set up a brain environment that is prone to mood disorders and even psychosis. When we start to understand how trauma(s) can set one up for increased emotional and mood challenges, then it starts to beg the question of how we approach mental illness, where we can start, and where we can try to prevent it from occurring in the first place.

What Now?

Why are things like child abuse or domestic violence so hidden from society? While we may "enjoy" watching movies with violence or watching the media with their guts and gore approach, actually taking on trauma personally or with a loved one is a very different animal. Families and friends like homeostasis. Conflict and separations are painful and hard to repair. Unfortunately, we also live with a human body conditioned to "hear no evil, see no evil, speak no evil," which makes talking about trauma with loved ones so challenging. We see this in psychology experiments that confirm the existence of a "bystander effect." The bystander effect is where multiple people witness a terrible event occurring, like an accident or violence, but because the people see each other and know that others have seen the incident, they fall into a "bystander" mode, which makes the person pass the responsibility of committing to action to help to another person. This tends to leave people who are being abused in the dark about their trauma because the tendency is to simply ignore it or not engage with it, especially if they know that other people know. Why do people sometimes take the side of the abuser, only to indirectly make the victim the perpetrator? As humans, to speak, acknowledge, and commit to action with the abused is to take on the burden of what trauma brings, which is disgust, anger, sadness, and anxiety. To take it on, the person is willing to alter or change their coping of trying to make the world look and fair. Some, if not most people, are not willing to make that much compromise, so they simply ignore the abused, or tell them not to tell anyone about it. This is incredibly common in families, unfortunately. The idea of having a family completely disintegrate from a child stating that a caregiver did something to them is truly overwhelming to many, who then just ignore it, especially when there is a significant amount of energy being put into the family already. We don't like to think of the world of being so evil, so cruel, and so unfair. This is why you'll see a statement like, "well, what was she wearing?" "Was she drunk at the time?" This is a way for us to soften the cruelty and injustice behind the trauma and to attribute "some fault" to both parties because this makes us feel better about ourselves and the world. But in the end, it discredits and puts the victim-centered stage, making it their responsibility to defend and face the trauma by having to explain it. Like a public defender trying to make you crack, this re-living and re-telling of the trauma and then being left alone leads to the isolation, mistrust, and injustice felt by abuse victims.

Victim blaming and isolating abused people needs to change if we are to ever make any headwind against the tragedy of trauma and mental illness. As social creatures, isolation is incredibly detrimental to us. The stigma with trauma and complete fear of being judged keep so many people in the dark, only for their body to manifest the horrendous event leading to unexplained anger or internalized body system failures that lead to chronic pain or autoimmune issues. We need to understand that people who experience trauma live in a dichotomy. They mistrust and want to protect themselves from others, but at the same time, they absolutely crave to be securely attached to a loved one who understands them and supports them. This dichotomy can create a world that is confusing to those who haven't been abused or traumatized, and it may appear "erratic." Taking a person's abuse claims seriously and doing the appropriate actions is crucial, especially when they are a child. Even when a child is abused, their reaching out and begging for help creates an opportunity for someone to be an adult role model who does what is right and supports the child and does everything to try and keep them safe. It may seem odd to not take a child seriously regarding any abuse, but surprisingly, many caregivers find themselves in very difficult situations when they are actually put in the position to take on abuse. Many don't know how to event begins, or even fathom the necessary actions to take place. What do you think you would do? Call police? Child Protective Services? While these are not bad ideas, anybody who has ever dealt with these systems to get help are usually met with very superficial investigations and odd laws that prevent further investigations into deeper matters.

This brings up another matter, and that is how the system handles abuse and traumatic events. Some of us have heard about the difficulties of going through the legal system to get any sort of justice for abuse. People who abuse typically do it in secrecy and for a reason, because most of the time authorities won't be able to put enough evidence forward. This is well known for anybody who works with rape victims. Only 1 in 10 rapes in the United States go to the authorities or the hospital. It's not hard to see why. Anytime someone is sexually assaulted, the first and foremost thought is typically to clean themselves. Without going into much detail but allowing imagination to run, bathing is a common first action of anyone who is sexually assaulted. Unfortunately, for investigative purposes, this eliminates quite a bit of evidence. But what does someone have to go through if they go to the emergency room? Rape kits, in theory, seem appropriate, and when they work, it's a very liberating experiencing for anyone who has been sexually assaulted. Unfortunately, rape kits are another trauma experience in themselves. One odd anomaly is that most rape kits are charged to the person still, with most costing over $1000. It is a deterrent to most.

Even if the decision to get a rape kit completed occurs, the process could be brutal. The process can take upwards of 4 hours and targets all the areas where the trauma occurred. This leads to the victim having to relive the trauma via strangers focusing on the parts that have been damaged. One such patient I had stated that she was raped by a man at a "college Halloween party." Even though she was having fun with her friends, dancing, and drinking alcohol, she never expected that a guy she never met would ask her to help him find the bathroom. She explained her experience with her rape kit during a session with me to give me a picture of "why" she would never go through this experience again. After being told not to wash anything off, she was left for 3 hours with his semen on her. Because the rape included forced oral copulation, she said that she could "taste" him for hours, and all she focused on was using mouthwash or brushing her teeth, but this wasn't allowed due to the evidence gathering process. Because traumatic experiences make your memory center go into complete disarray to protect you from the details, having to retell her story over and over not only made her look unbelievable, but also solidified the experience in her brain over and over with having to think of the experience. The kit was collected. And as of now (2019), it's been two years, and the kit has not been processed. This is a travesty of any sense of the word "justice." It's not fair to speculate the idea that she was "drinking alcohol" and was "dressed in a provocative costume," meaning to some that she was asking to be a target, which seemingly creates an odd justification for such an act to some. That's likened to saying that you were driving 48 miles an hour in a 45 mile per hour zone, and you got t-boned by a person who ran a red light and then pointing out that going 45 miles per hour was a huge contributor to the accident. The dialogue simply needs to change, and it needs to come from a place where people acknowledge that trauma and violence occur much more than we are comfortable to admit, even to our loved ones.

We need to pressure officials to take sexual assaults and rape kits more seriously. Even though funding may be an issue with child protective services and other agencies serviced to protect the abused, allowing broader policies to allow more serious investigations are crucial. So many child abuses fly under the radar because of our need for a more sensitive system to pick up on reports and actually investigate them appropriately. Anyone who works in child protective services, I think, would agree with me that they are usually inundated with cases with very little power to do anything. Rape kits need to be taken seriously and actually processed to investigate potential suspects. Research shows time and time again that an abuser will continue to abuse victim after victim.

More fundamentally, we need to move toward the education of the general public of the developmental effects of trauma on children. It's amazing how fast the public learned of PTSD with combat veterans and how fast most grasp their suffering (which is completely valid!). Why can't we do this for other types of traumatic events? Especially with the growing evidence that trauma can not only be a factor in mental illness but lead to generations of trauma being passed down like inheritances that are hidden in the closet. For Christians, this was seen as something similar to "generational sin," that is, the sins of one generation pass to the next generations. This could make sense to a population who didn't know how trauma affects the brain and how it interacts with others. "She was a prostitute and now look, her daughter hears voices and is doing drugs." Understanding the trauma model, we can understand how this can occur. Traumatized victims are not a morality case. Once morality verdicts get involved, shame and guilt grow. We need to move to a place where we accept what is, without odd excuses to minimize the true experience. This requires us to move to a place where we begin to take traumatic events seriously, and when we take action, the systems we vote for (and pay for) actually take the seriousness to do what is right for our human nature. To live is to experience suffering, but to live is also to strive to limit its grasp on our humanity

14

CONCLUSION

"This too shall pass."
- Persian adagy

Arming yourself with knowledge is always a key factor in getting the results we desire. My goal for this book was to provide information on the array of conditions and treatments found in mental health. Hopefully, it was a resource to provide some depth and understanding to a world that is often confusing and difficult to manage. Mental health faces a lot of battles and struggles ahead. Simply getting any consensual understanding of mental illnesses is a goal we can only dream of at this time. Differences of opinion are not bad per se! But they can create a lot of misinformation and poor understanding in a time when good and solid information, along with understanding, is crucial. We face a mental health system that is the most broken of systems in the United States, and all to no fault of the person suffering. Often with great frustration, families, and people who have mental conditions struggle to find their path to treatment and recovery. Knowing the complexities of the mind and our unique characteristics, will we ever have a genuine consensus on mental health? This is a true and provocative question, and we need to come to grips with it. Fundamentally, mental illness provides a raw look into our humanity. To suffer, to feel pain, to struggle are all human experiences. For many, simply looking into the suffering is too much to bear and giving simple answers to complex issues then prospers. Being able to embrace ourselves and others who suffer is challenging, but ultimately the best medicine there can be for mental illness and for any well-being.

Learning What We Can and Cannot Control

Some of the best advice in the mental health world is understanding what you can control and cannot control. What does this mean? When engaging in treatment and advocating for care, it's important to know and own the things you can do to help reach recovery, while letting go of what we ultimately have no control over because of the stage the world is in currently. This isn't to say not to strive for optimal care and opportunities, but it's just as important to understand that if you cannot control some aspect of mental health treatment or condition, that doesn't indicate a weakness or indifference. This can pertain to obtaining a type of treatment that you feel will work well for a loved one, but then have the loved one reject it. Or maybe trying to have a loved one try a new medication only to have them stop all their medications. Addiction knows this notion very well. The serenity prayer has the wise statement, "to grant me the serenity to accept the things I cannot change, the courage to change the things I can, and the wisdom to know the difference." We can't force people to do treatment (unless under extraordinary circumstances), and we don't typically get far when people are forced to do something they don't want to do. Humans have a primal instinct to be in control and make decisions for themselves. The frustrations that come when two people are trying to gain control on two different terms can be gut-wrenching, heart aching, and frustrating. Being able to accept where you have control and (more difficult) accepting what you don't have control over allows you to feel more content, along with putting energy into the appropriate channels.

CONCLUSION

Finding Your Path

No set combination of mental health treatments is a panacea for all. As stated before, our minds are all unique and different. We should expect that conditions with the mind are unique and different as well. That is not to say that some similar treatments are used to treat certain conditions. I couldn't be in my position if I believed that. But this is more to the core of our humanity. Of course, people with schizophrenia will ultimately need medications for the rest of their lives (granted they accept to take them), and having bipolar disorder without any medications is downright, leading to a life of extreme ups and downs in a world that generally won't tolerate it. Some can do psychotherapy for their panic disorder and never touch medications and be panic-free after the 6th session for the rest of their lives. Finding the right combination of treatments and connections is crucial to anyone's mental health functioning. Some of the more important factors include the basics of living, good quality sleep, a healthy diet, and good social connections are crucial to lay down a foundation for quality of life. Neglect any one of these and any mental health treatment may not be able to help with much. For some, hiking, being in nature, doing a sport, quilting, reading, skydiving, and more can be a hobby that keeps their mental health quality alive. Ultimately, it is your path and your destination to feel happy and to have great well-being. No one will do it for you, and yes, it is a lot of trial and error, and tears, and anguish, but any pursuit that is in line with your mental health goals and your vitality is worth every ounce of energy we have. I hope this book has served you well on this journey and to many journeys to come.

Safe journey on....

RESOURCES

National Alliance on Mental Illness (NAMI) is one of the premier mental health organizations in the United States. Their work focuses on mental health awareness, support, and policy development. This is a great resource for FREE mental health support groups in your community. Including family support groups.

https://www.nami.org/

Mental Health America (MHA) is a leader in mental health information, support and is driven to address many mental health needs in the United States. Go here to do free screenings, learn information about mental health conditions and treatment, and see what policies are being advocated for the future of mental health.

http://www.mentalhealthamerica.net/

Psychology Today is well known as a pop psychology magazine, but its real power is the listings of therapists and prescribers. See many providers in your area based on their specialties, costs, and even insurance covered.

https://www.psychologytoday.com/us

The Brain and Behavior Research Foundation is the premier mental health research funding organizations in the United States. Want to see and keep up with some of the greatest research on mental health? Feeling generous? They are one of the best mental health non-profits to donate too. Money given is spent 100% on mental health research.

https://www.bbrfoundation.org/

Good Therapy is a great site that discusses all things psychotherapy. Their search function to find a therapist is easy and straightforward, with ways to filter your results based on your needs.

https://www.goodtherapy.org/

Self-Management and Recovery Training (SMART) Recovery, a non-12 step approach, provides group support for any addiction. Many of the techniques are evidenced-based (CBT and emotional distress tolerance). These groups are FREE and can be done in person or ONLINE.

https://www.smartrecovery.org/

The Depression and Bipolar Support Alliance (DBSA) is a wonderful support group for those with depression or bipolar (although other mental conditions can attend). These are free and led by a peer leader. They have groups all over the nation and also online groups. Just remember: this is not a group to discuss medications (a topic they will redirect you from), but to work on skills and advocacy for your mental condition.

https://www.dbsalliance.org/

12-Step (Alcoholics Anyonymous/Narcotics Anonymous/ more) is one of the oldest addiction groups, 12 step is the basis of Alcoholics Anonymous, Narcotics Anonymous, Marijuana Anonymous, Overeaters Anonymous and many more. The 12 traditions are the backbone of the groups and have helped millions of people with addiction.

https://www.aa.org/

See more update resources at www.virtuesofmentalhealth.com/mental-health-resources

REFERENCES

Álvarez-Jiménez, M., Parker, A. G., Hetrick, S. E., Mcgorry, P. D., & Gleeson, J. F. (2009). Preventing the second episode: A Systematic review and meta-analysis of psychosocial and pharmacological trials in first-episode psychosis. *Schizophrenia Bulletin*, 37(3), 619–630. doi: 10.1093/ schbul/sbp129

Amador, X. (2007).*I am not sick: how to help someone with mental illness accept treatment.* Peconic: Vida Press.

American Foundation for Suicide Prevention. (2019, April 16). Suicide statistics. Retrieved from https://afsp.org/about-suicide/suicide-statistics/

American Psychiatric Publishing. (2013). *Diagnostic and statistical manual of mental disorders*(5th ed.). Arlington.

Banks, S. (2010, August 7). The crack epidemic's toxic legacy. Retrieved from https://www.latimes.com/archives/la-xpm-2010-aug-07-la-me-banks-20100807-story.html.

Bayard, M., McIntyre, J., Hill, K., & Woodside, J. (2004, March 15). Alcohol withdrawal syndrome. Retrieved from https://www.aafp.org/afp/2004/0315/p1443.html.

Belsky, J., & Pluess, M. (2009). Beyond diathesis stress: Differential susceptibility to environmental influences. *Psychological Bulletin*, 135(6), 885–908. doi: 10.1037/a0017376

Beronio, K., Po, R., Skopec, L., & Glied, S. (2013). Affordable Care Act expands mental health and substance use disorder benefits and Federal Parity Protections for 62 million Americans. Retrieved from https://aspe.hhs.gov/report/affordable-care-act-expands mental-health-and-substance-use-disorder-benefits-and-federal-parity protections-62-million-americans

Bhattacharyya, S., & Schoeler, T. (2013). The effect of cannabis use on memory function: An update. *Substance Abuse and Rehabilitation, 4,* 11–27. doi: 10.2147/sar.s25869

Bowen Center. (n.d.). Eight concepts. Retrieved from https://thebowencenter.org/theory/eight-concepts

Burns, D. D. (2007). *When panic attacks: the new, drug-free anxiety therapy that can change your life.* New York: Morgan Road Books. Castle, D. J. (2013). Cannabis and psychosis: What causes what? *F1000 Medicine Reports,5.* doi: 10.3410/m5-1

Centers for Disease Control and Prevention. (2019). About the CDC-Kaiser ACE study. Retrieved from https://www.cdc.gov/violenceprevention/child-abuseandneglect/acestudy/about.html

Centers for Disease Control and Prevention. (n.d.). Map of cigarette use among adults. Retrieved from https://www.cdc.gov/statesystem/cigaretteuseadult.html

Center for Substance Abuse Treatment. (2005). *Medication-assisted treatment for opioid addiction in opioid treatment programs.* Rockville, MD.

Center for Substance Abuse Treatment. (2014). *Treatment for stimulant use disorders.* Rockville, MD.

Cherry, K. (2019, July 15). How hypnosis is used in psychology. Retrieved from https://www.verywellmind.com/what-is-hypnosis-2795921

Clark, W., Welch, S. N., Berry, S. H., Collentine, A. M., Collins, R., Lebron, D., & Shearer, A. L. (2013). California's historic effort to reduce the stigma of mental illness: The Mental Health Services Act. *American Journal of Public Health, 103*(5), 786–794. doi: 10.2105/ajph.2013.301225

Felitti, V. J., Anda, R. F., Nordenberg, D., Williamson, D. F., Spitz, A. M., Edwards, V., … Marks, J. S. (1998). Relationship of childhood abuse and household dysfunction to many of the leading causes of death in adults. *American Journal of Preventive Medicine, 14*(4), 245–258. doi: 10.1016/s0749-3797(98)00017-8

Foote, J., Wilkens, C., Kosanke, N., & Higgs, S. (2014). *Beyond addiction: How science and kindness help people change: A guide for families.* New York, NY: Scribner.

Frances, R. (2012). "A Disease Like Any Other"? A decade of change in public reactions to schizophrenia, depression, and alcohol dependence. *Yearbook of Psychiatry and Applied Mental Health, 167*(11), 117–118. doi: 10.1016/j.ypsy.2011.07.010

Gahlinger, P. M. (2004). *Illegal drugs: A complete guide to their history, chemistry, use and abuse.* New York: Plume.

Galanti, G. A. (2015). *Caring for patients from different cultures*(5th ed.). Philadelphia: University of Pennsylvania Press.

Grady, S. E., Marsh, T. A., Tenhouse, A., & Klein, K. (2017). Ketamine for the treatment of major depressive disorder and bipolar depression: A review of the literature. *Mental Health Clinician, 7*(1), 16–23. doi: 10.9740/mhc.2017.01.016

Guilford Press. (2013). *Motivational interviewing: Helping people change*(3rd ed.). New York, NY.

Halter, M. J. (2014). *Varcarolis foundations of psychiatric-mental health nursing: A clinical approach*(7th ed.). St. Louis, MO: Elsevier.

Hare, R. D. (1999).*Without conscience: The disturbing world of the psychopaths among us*. New York, NY: The Guilford Press.

Harris, G. (2011, March 5). Talk doesn't pay, so psychiatry turns instead to drug therapy. Retrieved from https://www.nytimes.com/2011/03/06/health/policy/06doctors.html.

Harris, R. (2019).*Act made simple: An easy-to-read primer on acceptance and commitment therapy*. Oakland, CA: New Harbinger Publications, Inc.

Hart, W., Tortoriello, G. K., & Richardson, K. (2018). Are personality disorder traits ego-syntonic or ego-dystonic? Revisiting the issue by considering functionality. *Journal of Research in Personality, 76*, 124–128. doi: 10.1016/j.jrp.2018.08.001

Herman, J. L. (2015). *Trauma and recovery: The aftermath of violence, from domestic abuse to political terror*. New York: Basic Books.

Jamison, K. R. (2001). *Night falls fast: Understanding suicide*. London: Pan Macmillan.

Junger, S. (2017).*Tribe*. Boston, MA: Fourth Estate Ltd.

Kapur, S. (2003). Psychosis as a state of aberrant salience: A framework linking biology, phenomenology, and pharmacology in schizophrenia. *American Journal of Psychiatry, 160*(1), 13–23. doi: 10.1176/appi.ajp.160.1.13

Kellner, C. H., & Patel, S. B. (2018, August 24). The role of ECT in the suicide epidemic. Retrieved from https://www.psychiatrictimes.com/electroconvulsive-therapy/role-ect-suicide-epidemic.

Kessler, R. C., Amminger, G. P., Aguilar-Gaxiola, S., Alonso, J., Lee, S., & Ustun, T. B. (2007). Age of onset of mental disorders: A review of recent literature. *Current Opinion in Psychiatry, 20*(4), 359–364. doi: 10.1097/yco.0b013e32816ebc8c

Korb, A. (2019). *The upward spiral: using neuroscience to reverse the course of depression, one small change at a time.* Oakland, CA: New Harbinger Publications, Inc.

Kreisman, J. J., & Straus, H. (2010). *I hate you—don't leave me: Understanding the borderline personality.* New York, NY: Penguin.

Lamb, M. (2019, August 20). An overview of group therapy. Retrieved from https://www.verywellmind.com/what-is-group-therapy-2795760.

Learning, L. (n.d.). Lifespan development. Retrieved from https://courses.lumenlearning.com/wm-lifespandevelopment
 /chapter/the-graying-population-and-life-expectancy/.

Luhrmann, T. M. (2001). *Of two minds: An anthropologist looks at American psychiatry.* New York: Vintage Books.

Madhusoodanan, S., & Ting, M. B. (2014, January 15). Managing psychosis in patients with Alzheimer disease. Retrieved from https://www.psychiatrictimes.com/geriatric-psychiatry/managing-psychosis-patients-alzheimer-disease.

Mason, P. T., & Kreger, R. (2007). *Stop walking on eggshells.* Oakland, CA: New Harbinger Publications.

Maté, G. (2009). *In the realm of hungry ghosts: Close encounters with addiction.* Toronto: Vintage Canada.

Masterson, J. F. (2015). *The personality disorders through the lens of attachment theory and the neurobiologic development of the self: A clinical integration.* Phoenix, AZ: Zeig, Tucker & Theisen, Inc.

Mayo Clinic. (2018, November 1). Hypnosis. Retrieved from https://www.mayoclinic.org/tests-procedures/hypnosis/about/pac-20394405

Meeks, T. W. (2019, March 4). Antipsychotics in dementia: Beyond 'black-box' warnings. Retrieved from https://www.mdedge.com/psychiatry/article/63168/antipsychotics-dementia-beyond-black-box-warnings.

Merz, B. (2016, December 13). Benzodiazepine use may raise risk of Alzheimer's disease. Retrieved from https://www.health.harvard.edu/blog/benzodiazepine-use-may-raise-risk-alzheimers-disease-201409107397.

Micozzi, M. S. (2015). *Fundamentals of complementary and alternative medicine.* Philadelphia: Saunders.

Miller, A. (2008).*The drama of the gifted child: The search for the true self.* New York: BasicBooks.

Millon, T., Grossman, S. D., Meagher, S. E., & Millon, C. N. (2004). *Masters of the mind: Exploring the story of mental illness from ancient times to the new millennium.* Hoboken, NJ: Wiley.

Millon, T., Millon, C. M., Meagher, S. E., Grossman, S. D., & Ramnath, R. (2004). *Personality disorders in modern life*(2nd ed.). Hoboken, NJ: John Wiley & Sons.

Monico, N., & Thomas, S. (2019). Alcoholics Anonymous (AA) & the 12 steps. Retrieved from https://www.alcohol.org/alcoholics-anonymous/#12-steps-of-aa—-what-are-they

Murphy, R., Nutzinger, D., Paul, T., & Leplow, B. (2004). Conditional-associative learning in eating disorders: A comparison With OCD. *Journal of Clinical and Experimental Neuropsychology, 26*(2), 190–199. doi: 10.1076/j-cen.26.2.190.28091

Naessén, S., Carlström, K., Garoff, L., Glant, R., & Hirschberg, A. L. (2006). Polycystic ovary syndrome in bulimic women – An evaluation based on the new diagnostic criteria.*Gynecological Endocrinology, 22*(7), 388–394. doi: 10.1080/09513590600847421

Najavits, L. M. (2003). *Seeking safety: a treatment manual for Ptsd and substance abuse.* New York, NY, etc.: The Guilford Press.

National Eating Disorders Association. (n.d.). Insurance & legal issues. Retrieved from https://www.nationaleatingdisorders.org/learn/general-information/insurance.

New York-Presbyterian. (n.d.). Understanding BPD. Retrieved from https://www.nyp.org/bpdresourcecenter/borderline-personality-disorder/understanding-bpd

Newport, F. (2019, September 4). In U.S., estimate of LGBT population rises to 4.5%. Retrieved from https://news.gallup.com/poll/234863/estimate-lgbt-population-rises.aspx.

Perry, B. D., & Szalavitz, M. (2017). *The boy who was raised as a dog: And other stories from a child psychiatrists notebook: What traumatized children can teach us about loss, love, and healing.* New York: Basic Books.

Platt, M. G., Luoma, J. B., & Freyd, J. J. (2016). Shame and dissociation in survivors of high and low betrayal trauma. *Journal of Aggression, Maltreatment & Trauma, 26*(1), 34–49. doi: 10.1080/10926771.2016.1228020

Preston, J. D. (2015). *Child and adolescent clinical psychopharmacology made simple, 3rd edition.* New Harbinger Publications.

Sadock, B. J., Sadock, V. A., & Ruiz, P. (2015). *Kaplan & Sadock's synopsis of psychiatry: Behavioral sciences/clinical psychiatry*(11th ed.). Philadelphia: Wolters Kluwer.

Savage, D., & Miller, T. (2016). *It gets better: Coming out, overcoming bullying, and creating a life worth living.* New York: Penguin Books.

Shapiro, F. (2014). The role of eye movement desensitization and reprocessing (emdr) therapy in medicine: Addressing the psychological and physical symptoms stemming from adverse life experience. *The Permanente Journal,* 71–77. doi: 10.7812/tpp/13-098

Shaughnessy, M. J. (2017). Integrative literature review on shame. *Nursing Science Quarterly,31*(1), 86–94. doi: 10.1177/0894318417741120

Simon, G. K. (2016). *In sheep's clothing: Understanding and dealing with manipulative people.* Marion, MI: Parkhurst Brothers, Inc., Publishers.

SMART Recovery. (2019). Addiction help for individuals: Alternative to AA. Retrieved from https://www.smartrecovery.org/individuals/?_ga=
   2.96656605.393562001.1570495288-1835558234.1570495288

Sobel, S. V. (2012). *Successful psychopharmacology: Evidence-based treatment solutions for achieving remission.* New York: W.W. Norton & Co.

Solomon, A. (2016).*The noonday demon.* London: Vintage Publishing.

Stahl, S. M., & Grady, M. M. (2017). *Prescriber's guide: Stahl's essential psychopharmacology.* Cambridge, United Kingdom: Cambridge University Press.

Stahl, S. M., & Muntner, N. (2017). *Stahl's essential psychopharmacology: Neuroscientific basis and practical applications*(4th ed.). Cambridge: Cambridge University Press.

Stern, A. P. (2018, February 23). Transcranial magnetic stimulation (TMS): Hope for stubborn depression. Retrieved from https://www.health.harvard.edu/blog/transcranial-magnetic-stimulation-for-depression-2018022313335.

Stieff, F. V. (2011). *Brain in balance: Understanding the genetics and neurochemistry behind addiction and sobriety.* San Francisco: Canyon Hill Pub.

Szalavitz, M. (2017). *Unbroken brain: A revolutionary new way of understanding addiction.* Picador USA.

The Management of Posttraumatic Stress Disorder Work Group. (2017). *Va/DoD clinical practice guideline for the management of posttraumatic stress disorder and acute stress disorder: Guideline summary.* Washington, D.C.

Thompson, S. R., & Dobbins, S. (2017). The applicability of resilience training to the mitigation of trauma-related mental illness in military personnel. *Journal of the American Psychiatric Nurses Association, 24*(1), 23–34. doi: 10.1177/1078390317739957

Valiente-Gómez, A., Moreno-Alcázar, A., Treen, D., Cedrón, C., Colom, F., Pérez, V., & Amann, B. L. (2017). EMDR beyond PTSD: A systematic literature review. *Frontiers in Psychology, 8.* doi: 10.3389/fpsyg.2017.01668

van der Kolk, B. A.(2015). *The body keeps the score: brain, mind, and body in the healing of trauma*. NY, NY: Penguin Books.

Walker, E. F., & Diforio, D. (1997). Schizophrenia: A neural diathesis-stress model. *Psychological Review, 104*(4), 667–685. doi: 10.1037//0033-295x.104.4.667

Wesson, D. R., & Ling, W. (2003). The clinical opiate withdrawal scale (COWS). *Journal of Psychoactive Drugs, 35*(2), 253–259. doi: 10.1080/02791072.2003.10400007

Wheeler, K. (2014). *Psychotherapy for the advanced practice psychiatric nurse: A how-to guide for evidence-based practice*(2nd ed.). New York: Springer Publishing Company.

World Health Organization. (2019). Dementia. Retrieved from https://www.who.int/news-room/fact-sheets/detail/dementia

World Health Organization. (2019). Depression. Retrieved from https://www.who.int/news-room/fact-sheets/detail/depression

World Health Organization. (2019, July 26). Tobacco. Retrieved from https://www.who.int/news-room/fact-sheets/detail/tobacco

Yearwood, E. L., Pearson, G. S., & Newland, J. A. (2012). *Child and adolescent behavioral health: A resource for advanced practice psychiatric and primary care practitioners in nursing*. Chichester, West Sussex, UK: Wiley-Blackwell.

Zerwas, S., & Bulik, C. M. (2011). Genetics and epigenetics of eating disorders. *Psychiatric Annals, 41*(11), 532–538. doi: 10.3928/00485713-20111017-06

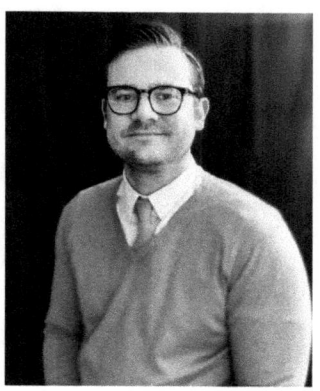

About the Author

Douglas Wagemann II MSN, PMHNP-BC, is a Board Certified Psychiatric Mental Health Nurse Practitioner (PMHNP). He currently practices in California and has mental health experience with Parole substance abuse services, community outpatient homeless treatment, VA PTSD clinic, and inpatient experience in forensics, substance abuse, severe mental illness, geriatric psychiatry, and crisis stabilization. He also teaches psychiatric nursing and community health nursing. He enjoys writing and is the creator of the Virtues of Mental Health blog.

www.ingramcontent.com/pod-product-compliance
Lightning Source LLC
Chambersburg PA
CBHW070912030426
42336CB00014BA/2384